*THE COLUMBIA
UNIVERSITY COLLEGE OF
DENTAL MEDICINE,
1916–2016*

The Columbia University College of Dental Medicine, 1916–2016

A Dental School on University Lines

Allan J. Formicola

Columbia University Press   New York

Columbia University Press
Publishers Since 1893
New York   Chichester, West Sussex
cup.columbia.edu

Library of Congress Cataloging-in-Publication Data
Names: Formicola, Allan J., author.
Title: The Columbia University College of Dental Medicine, 1916-2016 :
    a dental school on university lines / Allan J. Formicola.
Description: New York : Columbia University Press, [2016] |
    Includes bibliographical references and index.
Identifiers: LCCN 2016014648 | ISBN 9780231180887 (cloth : alk. paper)
Subjects: | MESH: Columbia University. Dental School. | Columbia University.
    College of Dental Medicine. | Columbia University. School of Dental and
    Oral Surgery. | Schools, Dental—history | Education, Dental—history |
    History of Dentistry | History, 20th Century | History, 21st Century |
    New York City
Classification: LCC RK76 | NLM WU 19 AN7 | DDC 617.60071/1—dc23
LC record available at https://lccn.loc.gov/2016014648

Columbia University Press books are printed on permanent and durable acid-free paper.
Printed in the United States of America

c 10 9 8 7 6 5 4 3 2 1

Cover design: Jason Gabbert
Cover image: © Carol M. Highsmith

This book is dedicated to the faculty and leaders who mentored generations of students over the past hundred years. Their efforts have translated the founding document, A Dental School on University Lines, *into the Columbia University College of Dental Medicine we know today.*

Contents

Foreword

This book celebrates the 100th anniversary of the College of Dental Medicine. It traces the legacy of its founders and early faculty, their challenges and strengths, and the dental school's long relationship with the medical school. It is a unique story, one that encourages the dental school's leadership, faculty, and graduates to continually revisit and revise its programs to maintain its excellence in the field and its strength within the university system. Indeed, the book rekindles thinking about the purpose of the institution and its current culture along with its traditions.

In a larger sense, the book also shows how dentistry fits into the medical field. The diseases and deformities of the orofacial complex affect the entire body. From the school's very beginning, the university, the medical school, and the dental school's founders recognized that the education for those who treat these conditions must be at the same level as those who treat medical diseases and conditions. The founding document stated it this way: that the requirements for admission to the School of Dentistry "shall be the same as those for admission to the Medical School and whose students shall then pursue a four-year course, the first two years of which will be almost identical with the first two years of the course in Medicine." This history demonstrates the determination of the leadership at all levels of the university over the past 100 years to live up to that statement.

The dental school and school of medicine share a long and close history. Columbia University emerged from King's College, a pre-Revolutionary educational institution founded in 1754. Columbia had already established a medical faculty in 1767 when it merged with he independent College of Physicians and Surgeons (P&S) in 1813. By 1891 P&S was fully incorporated into Columbia University.

Just seven years later in 1898, a number of leading dentists in New York City approached the University to establish a dental school as well. There was little interest and willingness at that time to establish a dental school. It took until 1916, during the presidency of Nicholas Murray Butler, for the University to act to include dentistry as one of its schools.

Samuel Lambert, dean of P&S, chaired the committee that worked with leading dentists and William J. Gies, PhD, a biochemist at P&S, to prepare the founding document of the new dental school, entitled *A Dental School on University Lines*. The essence of its guidelines was based on the notion that the dental school be closely tied to the medical school. At its inception in 1916 the dental school shared facilities in the medical school building on Fifty-Ninth Street. Then in 1928, both the medical and dental schools moved to the newly constructed Columbia–Presbyterian Medical Center, forming the first complete medical campus in the world.

Allan Formicola willingly took on the task of preparing this history. He served as dean of the School of Dental and Oral Surgery for almost one-quarter of its 100-year history, bringing the school into the twenty-first century. His longevity in the position provided him with a deep understanding of the University and the Medical Center in which the dental school is set. This narrative of the school's history draws heavily from the written records available in the Archives and Special Collections of the Medical Center and University libraries. Formicola also spent a significant amount of time collecting stories from alumni about their student days to enliven the text.

It is important to reflect on an institution's history. This book links the past years of the School of Dental and Oral Surgery's with the currently renamed College of Dental Medicine. It shows that the founding document still remains the guiding principle for dentistry at Columbia University and the Columbia University Medical Center.

Lee Goldman
Dean of the Faculties of
Health Sciences and Medicine

Christian Stohler
Dean
College of Dental Medicine

Preface

In August of 2013, the newly appointed dean of the Columbia University College of Dental Medicine, Christian Stohler, invited me to write the history of the school to commemorate the 100th anniversary of its founding. I was happy to accept because I have always been intrigued with the role that Columbia played in the development of dental education in the United States in the early part of the twentieth century. The research for the book would provide me with the opportunity to delve deeply into that history. When I became dean in 1978, much of the school's history had been forgotten. It was therefore with great enthusiasm that I took on the task of preparing this history so that it would be remembered and passed on to future generations.

In preparing this book, it was important that the history be obtained from primary sources. The Archives and Special Collections at the Augustus C. Long Library on the Medical Center campus and at the Butler Library on the Morningside campus of Columbia University contain a trove of documents related to the founding of the dental school and its progress over the past century. They include records and files from the school's deans and the vice presidents for health science offices going back to the 1890s. Their formal reports, letters, and memorabilia provided the majority of the information for the book. In addition, interviews with key individuals such as faculty, students, and alumni were used to enrich the material from historical documents.

History came alive for me through contacts with family members of the founders—William J. Gies and the Dunning brothers—and the son of one of its legendary deans—Alfred Owre. Those contacts provided me with a deep appreciation and understanding of the important contributions made by these individuals and others to establish the Columbia University Dental School.

The history of the dental school at Columbia University is intimately intertwined with William J. Gies, William and Henry Dunning, and Alfred Owre. Gies was the author of the 1926 Carnegie Foundation report on the advancement of teaching, which is still credited today as the most important document in shaping dental schools in the United States and Canada. Gies was not a dentist but a biochemist at the Columbia University College of Physicians and Surgeons. He became interested in the field of dentistry in 1910, first through research on dental caries and later by working with leading New York dentists to prepare the school's founding document, *A Dental School on University Lines.*

That document and the dental school he helped found at Columbia became the model for Gies's recommendations in the Carnegie report. Its principles showed the way that dentistry should fit into the field of medicine and the nation's university system. Those principles are still relevant today. Similar issues regarding dentistry's position in the field of medicine and in the nation's university system have resurfaced. Throughout the text, therefore, reference is made to Gies's original educational principles.

William Bailey Dunning and Henry Sage Dunning were brothers and prominent dentists in New York City at the time of the founding of the school. William probably coauthored the founding document with Gies. Henry was an oral surgeon who raised funds to help establish the school. Both served on the faculty for many years.

Alfred Owre arrived as dean in 1927 and his task was to move the school from East Thirty-Fourth and Thirty-Fifth Streets to the Vanderbilt Clinic building on the newly completed Columbia University Medical Center campus on 168th Street. Owre had served as dean at the University of Minnesota before coming to Columbia. He became a controversial figure among the dentists in New York City because of his ideas about how dentistry should be integrated into medicine and how the dental school should operate.

I was fortunate to meet with family members of these four individuals in the 1980s. I was surprised one day when a second-year medical student at P&S came to my office asking whether or not her great-grandfather had something to do with the founding of the dental school. She was Marjorie Gies! Through her, I met her father, William (Bill) J. Gies II, a man who has shared remembrances, friendship, and service as we worked together on the American Dental Education Association's William J. Gies Foundation. Bill Gies provides the association's members with wonderful stories of his grandfather and in the process keeps the connection between William Gies and Columbia fresh in everyone's mind.

Similarly, I reconnected with the Dunning brothers' family. I received a call from James Dunning, a son of one of the distinguished founders of the Columbia University Dental School. Jim was an alumnus of the School of Dental and Oral Surgery (SDOS) and a former dean of the Harvard University School of Dental Medicine. He called to say that he came across some files from his father's (William Bailey Dunning) years at SDOS and wanted to donate them to Columbia. Along with the papers was also a gold cigar box that his uncle (Henry Sage Dunning) received from his oral surgery residents. Everything was put into the archives of the Augustus C. Long Library. Jim also made a donation to the school and, together, we created a symposium, the Dunning Symposium, in his family's name. Each year when we held the Dunning Symposium, Jim would attend and join in the discussion.

Alfred Owre's years at Columbia were difficult ones for him. That became apparent to me again in the 1980s during a visit from his son. One day my assistant, Letty Casillas, buzzed me to say that Alfred Owre was in the waiting room! I knew that was not possible, because he died in 1935 and this was the mid-1980s, but in walked his son of the same name, a man possibly in his seventies. He had come to Columbia looking for some of his father's papers so he could donate them to the University of Minnesota where a building was to be dedicated in his father's name. We talked and I learned that the son was a psychiatrist living in California and that he believed that his father was distressed for a long time about his treatment while at Columbia. I remember feeling uncomfortable and tried to assure him about his father's many positive contributions to the development of the school. A few years later, the associate dean, Norman Kahn, received a call saying that the caller had Alfred Owre's academic gown in her closet and would the school like to have it. Norman brought the gown to the school and I put it in the closet in the dean's office where it still sits today!

In so many different ways, the history of the dental school is fascinating. It includes insightful documents related to mergers with other schools and the story of a long and protracted controversy with the dental accrediting agency over the relationship between the dental school and the medical school and the Presbyterian Hospital. There is even the story of a "crazed" technician who murdered one of the deans at his desk in 1935!

With this as a background, how can knowing this history not evoke interest, pride, and continual support for the Columbia University College of Dental Medicine, "a dental school on university lines"?

Allan J. Formicola, DDS, MS
Dean Emeritus

Acknowledgments

I am indebted to the staff of the Archives and Special Collections at the Augustus C. Long Health Sciences Library of Columbia University. Stephen Novak, the head archivist, and Cameron Mitchell, library assistant, always made the dental school collection readily available and provided photocopies of important documents. Steve Novak provided good advice on early drafts of book chapters. I am also indebted to Ira Lamster, who drafted Chapter 4, "2001–2013: The New Millennium: The School of Dental and Oral Surgery Becomes the College of Dental Medicine," which covers the period of his deanship. Ronnie Myers also stepped up to the plate by drafting the last section of Chapter 4, which covers his period of interim deanship. The information needed for Chapter 5, "2013–2016 and Beyond: Plans for the Next 100 Years," was obtained from the chairs of the College of Dental Medicine's five sections, members of the administrative staff, the associate deans, and a group of enrolled students. I appreciate their cooperation in giving me that information.

Selecting the photographs and figures for the book was a monumental project. It required sorting through hundreds of photographs in the archives and school files. Melissa Welsh and Douglas McAndrew had the patience and persistence to assist me with this difficult task. Going from the initial draft to the final manuscript of the book required dedicated and talented editing. I was fortunate to have two talented individuals as editors. Jennifer Perillo, senior executive editor at the Columbia University Press, provided sage advice on ways to improve the initial draft of the manuscript and to include stories of graduates. I also appreciate her advice and suggestion to hire an editor to help me in moving from the initial draft to the final manuscript. This allowed me much-needed time to continue to do research. Nancy Bruning was the editor who accomplished multiple tasks, from ensuring that the chapters were placed in proper context to classic editing of the text and the stories from alumni to making sure that the photographs, illustrations, and appendixes added to the information and interest of the book to keeping us on schedule to finish the manuscript on time. She has been a delightful taskmaster!

Reading the drafts of chapters or the entire manuscript is an arduous task, requiring time and perseverance. I feel fortunate that a group of knowledgeable individuals reviewed the manuscript, improving it immeasurably. Thank you to Letty Moss-Salentijn, Martin Davis, Melissa Welsh, Louis Mandel, Marlene Klyvert, David Zegarelli, Ron Myers, Norman Kahn, and Zoila Nougerole for advice and comments on early drafts of the chapters. The final product was enriched by their suggestions. I am grateful for the support of my wife, Jo Renee Formicola, who has written four books and edited five other books. She continually encouraged me in the writing of this one and carefully read and critiqued various first drafts of the chapters. Her advice was always aimed at getting the drafts to become the best they could be.

I am grateful for the opportunity that Christian Stohler, the dean of the College of Dental Medicine, gave me to write this book. I value his confidence and trust in me and the chance to reconnect with the college in a vital new way through the preparation of the book. I am not an alumnus of Columbia University or the College of Dental Medicine. As an "outsider" arriving as dean, I have enjoyed hundreds of collegial relationships with the faculty, students, alumni, and staff of the school and with those up and down the line in the Medical Center and University. Over my thirty-three years at the university, of which twenty-three years were spent as dean, I awarded more than 2,000 degrees and certificates. In preparing this book I feel very much like an alumnus of the College of Dental Medicine and, in my own way, a member of the Columbia family. This is an exciting place with unlimited opportunities for all who seek them out. I still find it very exhilarating to be in its collegial environment. It has been a privilege to have researched and written this history.

Allan J. Formicola, DDS, MS
Dean Emeritus

*THE COLUMBIA
UNIVERSITY COLLEGE OF
DENTAL MEDICINE,
1916–2016*

Introduction

One hundred years is a long time in the life of an institution. This book commemorates the history of the College of Dental Medicine of Columbia University and traces the twists and turns in moving from its inception to its development as one of the premier dental schools in the world.

It is clear that the institution attracted a stellar group of early leaders. Several stand out. The giant among them, William J. Gies, was not a dentist but a biochemist at the College of Physicians and Surgeons. How Gies got involved in dentistry and attracted the best and the brightest of New York City dentists who collaborated with him to produce the school's visionary founding document, *A Dental School on University Lines*, is a unique story in the history of twentieth-century dentistry and in the history of Columbia University. Gies and his collaborators convinced Columbia University and the College of Physicians and Surgeons that a dental school was an important complement to the field of medical education, and that such a school should be part of the University.

The six chapters of this book record key periods in the school's development over the past 100 years and also provide a look into the future. The appendixes provide details and dates to supplement these earlier times. The documentation of the description of the history is contained in the bibliography.

Chapter 1 describes the first twenty-five years, from 1916 to 1941, and focuses on the challenges of a school trying to meet the vision of its creators. Their goal was to distinguish Columbia University's dental school from most other schools by its connection with medicine. The school they founded would become the model for dental schools across the nation. This chapter includes the controversy between two men, William Gies and Alfred Owre, both of whom shaped the institution with their divergent points of view on how the profession of dentistry should evolve in the nation and at Columbia University. It also tells the tale of the tragic murder of a dean killed by a crazed employee, which led to a major change in the relationship between the medical and dental schools and caused a protracted battle with the Council on Dental Education, the accrediting body.

Chapter 2 delves into the battle between Columbia's leadership and the dental accrediting body. These became difficult years for the school, from 1941 to 1978. The merger of the dental school with the medical school resulted in a loss of the school's accreditation. Several states in the Northeast refused to license Columbia graduates as a result, but Columbia prevailed in the end. The dental school adhered to its original vision after the school's early leadership and faculty retired. By the 1970s the leadership in the dental school was able to turn its attention to resolving other long-standing problems such as inadequate space for the school, a situation that stymied progress and caused additional accreditation issues.

Chapter 3 encompasses the last quarter of the twentieth century, 1978 to 2001, a period that saw rapid growth of the dental school. Many advances and a major shift in the financial relationship between New York State and the school characterize this era. In this chapter, the story of the school's great leap forward via a refocusing of its vision unfolds. The measures that grew out of that vision transformed the school and better integrated it with the Presbyterian Hospital and the other schools on the Medical Center and University campuses. Outreach to the northern Manhattan community expanded the school mission for the benefit of the underserved community that is its home. Accreditation issues were no longer an issue and the school improved its standing among peers.

Chapter 4 discusses the turnover into the twenty-first century, which brought further transitions for the school. Following the lead of the university and medical school, the dental school established a global outreach initiative. A name change for the school became a symbol of the shifting advances in dentistry from mostly a surgical field to a more medically oriented one. The school's name had evolved from the Columbia University Dental School to the School of Dental and Oral Surgery in 1923, and finally to the College of Dental Medicine in 2006, reflecting that shift. The research program expanded to joint programs with faculty from the schools of public health, the medical school and other units on the campus. Acquisition of new space for research endeavors enhanced those efforts. From 2001 to 2013 a continuing process of strategic growth occurred, while the school dealt with substantial financial issues.

Chapter 5 covers the period from 2013 to the present and beyond. Approaching its centennial year, the College of Dental Medicine stands poised for its next evolutionary phase. This chapter demonstrates how the school is attracting highly talented students and faculty and moving from the industrial age of dentistry into the digital one. It shows how the reorganization of teaching divisions is leading to a strengthening of programs in the current period as those sections gain greater programmatic and budgetary responsibility. Aligning the College of Dental Medicine's mission more closely with the other schools on the medical campus and with those of the University is leading to new opportunities for refining and bolstering the college.

One of the long-term problems plaguing the school from its earliest days was inadequate space. Now, however, the college appears to be at an important turning point, having acquired an additional floor in the Vanderbilt Clinic building. This building continues to be its historic home, as the school has been on 168th Street since it moved in 1928 from its adopted college's buildings on East Thirty-Fourth and Thirty-Fifth Streets.

Finally, Chapter 6 highlights many of the superb accomplishments of the students and alumni, as a reminder of the main purpose for academic institutions. The Columbia University Dental School inherited a large and diverse student population when it merged with the independent College of Dental and Oral Surgery in 1923. The graduates of the latter institution became alumni of Columbia University and helped solve the school's inherent struggle to attract and admit a diverse student body. This chapter relates the accomplishments of one graduate in particular, Elizabeth Delany, who became a national sensation at the age of 100. She and her sister wrote *Having Our Say*, a national best seller that became the subject of a play on Broadway and a television movie. She graduated in 1923 and practiced in Harlem, and she revealed in the book her struggle as an African American woman to receive equal treatment while in the dental school. Her story mirrors the fight for equality between the races in the United States until civil rights and affirmative action legislation in the 1960s and 1970s provided institutions with the tools to address the nation's long-standing refusal to admit students of color and women. This chapter picks up on how the dental school became involved in moving toward diversity in its student body and has emerged as a national leader in attracting students from underrepresented minority backgrounds today.

Dedicated educators create outstanding and loyal graduates. The Columbia University College of Dental Medicine alumni/ae are both. They have organized to assist the College in many ways by mentoring students, holding alumni events, becoming volunteer faculty, and raising funds. Graduates have provided leadership to the field and accomplished much. Throughout the chapters of the book, we provide stories of graduates as examples of the entire student body. Most of those stories were obtained from a randomly selected group of alumni/ae to illustrate points in the text. Other's stories, such as those of Seymour Lipton and Herbert Ferber, both internationally known sculptors, were selected to support the words of Alfred Owre, an early leader in the dental school, who recognized that dentistry would attract students from a diverse backgrounds in the arts as well as in the sciences. While it is impossible to recognize all of those who graduated from the SDOS/CDM in its 100-year history, we hope these stories bring to life the experiences of the school's students and faculty.

It is the author's hope that readers find this book interesting, informative, and inspiring. The College of Dental Medicine has the right to be proud. Leadership at all levels of the university helped to shape the College over the past 100 years. It has become truly "a dental school on university lines," just as Gies envisioned it, and adds to the rich environment of a world-class university.

Allan J. Formicola, DDS, MS
Dean Emeritus

CHAPTER ONE

1916–1941:
A Dental School on University Lines

To better understand the underpinnings and importance of the College of Dentistry, it helps to have a broad picture of the state of dentistry and dental education at the time of the school's founding.

In the late nineteenth and early twentieth centuries, dental decay (caries) was rampant in the population. There was little knowledge of the causes and prevention of the disease. The foot drill, invented in the early 1900s to remove carious lesions, was still in use until the latter part of the second decade. Amalgam became the most widely used material to restore teeth, although it was controversial due to its mercury content. Little attention was paid to the diagnosis and treatment of periodontal disease. Restorations were often placed on teeth with advanced periodontal infections without treating those infections. The focal infection theory of bodily disease caused by diseased or endodontically treated teeth and periodontal infections became the rationale to extract teeth rather than treat them.[1]

Dentistry was a profession whose practitioners were a product of apprenticeships rather than education in dental schools. In the early years of the twentieth century, many freestanding inferior proprietary dental schools existed in the United States. Dentistry was unregulated, which permitted unlicensed practitioners to prey on the public and provide unproven treatment and wholesale extraction of teeth. There were possibly 5,000 unlicensed dentists in New York City alone in the early 1900s, prompting a rise of concern in the press. This was an era of "advertising dentists," and "Painless Parker," one of the most notorious, claimed to have extracted 357 teeth in one day and made a necklace out of them.[2] Physicians, on the other hand, were uninterested in treating diseases of the oral cavity and mistakenly considered these diseases to be of local origin only, with little significance for overall health, and thought that extraction of teeth was the best treatment.

Eventually, there was a growing demand for ethical practitioners and a profession of dentistry based on a sound biomedical background. Calls to eliminate freestanding proprietary schools based on the apprenticeship model grew. Leaders in the profession encouraged universities to include dental schools under their aegis. In New York City, concern by leading practitioners of medicine and dentistry led to the first, unsuccessful attempt to found a dental school at Columbia University in 1898. A second, more successful effort had to wait until 1916.

THE FOUNDING

The complex chain of events that brought Columbia University, the College of Physicians and Surgeons, and the Presbyterian Hospital together to form the first complete medical center in the country set the stage for a similarly winding road for the dental school.

Building the Columbia University Medical Center

Columbia University, which was to become the home of the dental school, has a rich history in the nation's higher and medical education systems. The University traces its origins to King's College, founded in 1754, with a medical faculty established in 1767. After the Revolutionary War, the University was renamed Columbia University, and its medical faculty merged in 1814 with the College of Physicians and Surgeons (P&S), an independent medical college. In 1860 P&S became the medical faculty of the University, and in 1891 P&S was fully incorporated into the University. The dental school followed a similar path of incorporating an independent dental school into the Columbia University Dental School. The history of the dental school, the College of Dental Medicine (CDM), is based on a close relationship with the medical school. The year 1902 saw the appointment of Columbia's longtime president Nicholas Murray Butler, and with the appointment of Dr. Samuel Lambert as dean of the medical school in 1905, interest grew at Columbia to affiliate with the Presbyterian Hospital. Edward Harkness, who had joined the Presbyterian Hospital board, was the catalyst to bring together the Presbyterian Hospital with the medical school and the University to form the first complete medical center in the country. The twelve-acre Washington Heights site, purchased from the Vanderbilt family, was at that time the home of the New York Highlanders, later known as the New York Yankees. Plans to bring the medical school together with the Presbyterian Hospital were agreed upon in 1911. However, it would take until 1921 to work out the details and financing to actually begin the construction of the medical center, which opened in 1928. The negotiations were complicated, especially the raising of necessary funds, which turned out to be $11 million, or $152 million in 2014 dollars.

One cannot talk about the founding of the dental school without mentioning the Gies report. And one cannot understand the significance of the Gies report, *Dental Education in the United States and Canada*, without first reflecting on the Flexner report, *Medical Education in the United States and Canada*, which established the parameters of the Columbia University Medical Center.

The Flexner report was written by Abraham Flexner, an educator and graduate of Johns Hopkins University. His critique of 150 North American medical schools, published in 1910, caused a reform in medical education and ended an era of low-quality proprietary medical schools. He based many of his recommendations on what he had observed at the Johns Hopkins Medical Center. One of the major conclusions of his report was the importance of the hospital in the education of future physicians. Paramount in that relationship was the medical school's control over the clinical educational experiences of the third- and fourth-year medical students in the hospital. Flexner became a consultant on the formation of the Columbia University Medical Center and helped to shape the details of how the hospital and the University partnership was formed: basically the two institutions were connected at the hip through land, facilities, and the need for the hospital's physician staff to hold university appointments. As we will see, the Columbia University Dental School would also have its Flexner report—but it would become known as "the Gies report."

In 1916 Columbia University approved a proposal to establish a dental school. The founding document, *A Dental School on University Lines*, mapped out the future course for a dental school at Columbia as well as for dental schools in the United States and Canada. The founding document was written in 1916 by William J. Gies and a number of leading New York City dentists. Gies was a prolific researcher and faculty member in biochemistry at Columbia University; he would continue to be a major influence on the dental school.

The founding committee for the Columbia University Dental School was composed of twenty prestigious individuals, including the dean of the Columbia University College of Physicians and Surgeons, Samuel W. Lambert, and the chair of biochemistry, William J. Gies, as well as a group of sixteen of the most prominent dentists in New York City at the time, including Henry and William Dunning, William Jarvie, Leuman Waugh, and Henry Gillett. William Jarvie's brother, James, provided the first major gift for the dental school of $125,000 ($2.7 million in 2014 dollars). This sum was sufficient for the dental school to become part of the University and affiliated with the College of Physicians and Surgeons.

As set forth in the founding document, the committee's vision for the Columbia University Dental School was to be something new—a dental school on "university lines." In approving the committee's proposal, the trustees of the University indicated that the dental school was to be a school whose requirements for admissions were the same as those for the medical school, with the course of study in dentistry based on a four-year curriculum, of which the first two years would be "almost identical with the first two years of the course in medicine. The two last years would be given to special preparation for dentistry and dental surgery."[3] When the dental school opened for students in the 1916–1917 year, the course of study was five years in length, and dental students enrolled in the same basic science courses as the medical students. In the following year the course of study was reduced to four years. The courses included in the first two years were Anatomy, including Histology and Embryology, Biologic Chemistry, Physiology, Pathology, Pharmacology, the Practice of Medicine, and Surgery. In addition, dental students had preclinical courses in dentistry in the first two years and clinical courses in the third and fourth years. Until 1920, the few dental students who were enrolled attended all classes in the College of Physicians and Surgeons building on Fifty-Ninth Street. In 1920 a small annex to the medical school building and adjacent to the Vanderbilt Clinic opened for the dental school.

THE INFLUENCE OF WILLIAM J. GIES

It is impossible to describe the history of the College of Dental Medicine[4] without paying homage to William J. Gies, PhD (1872–1956). His involvement and expertise in dental research were crucial to the formation of the dental school at Columbia. At Yale University, where he was awarded the doctoral degree in 1897 at the age of 25, he became the assistant of the top professors, one of whom was world renowned in the field of physiological chemistry and also a lecturer at Columbia. Upon the recommendation of his Yale professors, Gies joined the Columbia medical school teaching

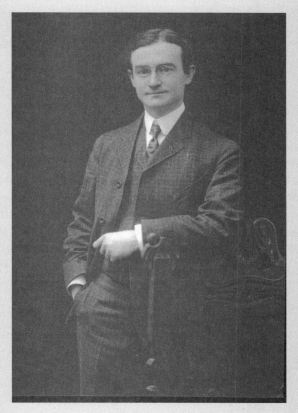

FIGURE 1.1 This photograph of William Gies, PhD, shows him as a young man, much as he appeared in the early decades of the twentieth century when he was getting involved with dentistry.

staff in 1898 and founded the first Department of Biological Chemistry in a medical school. Between 1903 and 1927, Gies published eight volumes of biological research papers, as well as textbooks in general, organic, and biological chemistry.

Gies was a prolific researcher and published many papers in dental journals. In fact, the *Journal of the Allied Dental Societies* in 1916 and 1917 alone carried seventeen of Gies's papers, several of which are listed in the bibliography for this chapter. Between 1909 and 1919 Gies, encouraged by the Dental Society of the State of New York (now the New York State Dental Society), conducted many far-reaching studies on the causes of dental caries and how to prevent the disease, a subject the society felt was being neglected in medical and dental schools. In a summary presentation to the Canadian Oral Prophylactic Association, Gies said his studies showed dental caries were the result of "acid as the destructive agent, bacteria the factors that make the acid, carbohydrate the substance that yields the acid." He further noted that in some individuals the bacteria could not grow in the mouth because "there is something in the saliva that is detrimental to them."[5] The latter concept was handed down in successive laboratories at the dental school through studies conducted by Irwin Mandel from the 1970s to the 1990s, which clearly demonstrated the protective role of saliva. The former studies on bacteria and carbohydrate as the destructive agents in dental caries were affirmed in the 1950s and beyond by respected microbiologists working in the field of dental research.

As a leader in dental research, Gies went on to found the *Journal of Dental Research* and the International Association of Dental Research in 1919. In 1923 he brought competing groups together to form the American Association of Dental Schools, which today is known as the American Dental Education Association. As a key member of the founders of the dental school, he recognized that the field of dentistry needed to substantially upgrade the education of its practitioners. He believed this was the only way dentistry could become part of the medical profession, and a profession based on a keen understanding of biological and pathological principles.

THE GIES REPORT

In 1919, nine years after the publication of the Carnegie Foundation's report on medical education by Abraham Flexner, the foundation approached William Gies to complete a similar study about education for dentistry. The Carnegie Foundation for the Advancement of Education understood that the same problems existed in dental schools in the first decade of the twentieth century as existed in medical schools. The foundation noted that there was still great controversy in how dentistry should be organized within the general field of medicine and whether dentistry was a separate profession from medicine or should be considered part of it. The foundation believed that the time was right to undertake a study on dental education to help answer these questions.

From 1919 to 1926, Gies compiled the most in-depth study of dental education ever undertaken. Known as "the Gies report," his report to the foundation was exhaustive. It covered the problems in the quality of care offered to the public as a result of poorly trained practitioners and defined the profession as closely related to medicine and as a partner to medicine in service to the public. The report laid out the requirements for dental schools to raise their student admissions standards and the necessity for full-time faculty devoted to pedagogy and scholarship. In coming to his findings, Gies visited every dental school in the United States and Canada, in total forty-eight schools—no easy task in the early part of the century. His report is credited with setting the standards needed for dental schools to become part of the university system in the United States and led to the closing of inferior freestanding technically oriented dental schools. Mergers of freestanding dental schools with universities became the norm. The principles and standards for dental schools in the 1926 report became codified into accreditation standards and have been upheld since then. They guide dental education today.

While Gies did not begin to work on the Carnegie Foundation report until 1919, his previous active work with the dental leaders in New York and with the leadership of Columbia University and the College of Physicians and Surgeons helped form his vision of dental education. His 1926 report therefore strongly reflects the philosophy and curriculum of the Columbia dental school. It called for two years of prerequisite course work for entrance into dental school. Columbia was the first school of dentistry in the nation to establish this requirement in 1919, seven years ahead of the report's publication. At the time, most states had a statutory requirement of a high school diploma or its equivalent for entry to dental schools. By the early 1920s, other dental schools followed Columbia's lead for college-level preparation for entrance to dental schools, and most states then began to require at least two years of college education for admission to dental school. The Gies report also called for a close affiliation of medical and dental education in the first two years, a full-time faculty dedicated to pedagogy and research, the incorporation of dental schools into the university system, and adequate financial and physical resources to meet its mission.

Gies viewed dentistry as an equal partner with medicine in providing for the health of the public and thought that educating practitioners required a close affiliation of medical and dental schools under the aegis of the university. Historically, medical schools had a low regard for dentistry, and the first attempt to include dental education at the medical school at the University of Maryland in the late 1830s was rejected. The medical faculty thought the subject of dentistry was unimportant. Several other medical schools, including those in New York, thought the same. The die had been cast! The Gies report recognized that as a consequence of dentistry being kept out of medical schools, dental schools emerging from the era of apprenticeships were established as independent schools. The exception was the dental school established in 1867 by Harvard University. It was the first dental school permanently established by a university. Gies defined dentistry as the oral specialty of medicine, but recognized that dentistry was a separate profession from medicine due to the traditions that had been built during the nineteenth and early twentieth centuries. He was able to translate the problems of the time concerning the profession of dentistry and how to reform it to educate "men and women to be wise and capable general practitioners, competent to begin a reliable independent service, and able to learn and also to grow steadily in proficiency and aspiration from experience and study."[6] With the publication of the Gies report, the battle over whether dentistry was a proper specialty of medicine was resolved.

The College of Dental Medicine at Columbia and Columbia University and its medical center were fortunate to have among their faculty a man of such great intellect and abilities. William J. Gies was truly an outstanding individual. He was the guiding light for the Columbia University Dental School, especially from 1916 through the 1930s. His direct influence on the school as part of the leadership and as a professor was felt until the time of his retirement in 1937 at the age of sixty-five. Today, when we celebrate the 100-year anniversary of the College of Dental Medicine, his influence over the school is still felt. Anyone wanting to learn more about the life of Dr. Gies should read his biography by Frank J. Orland.[7]

THE EARLY YEARS 1916–1928: LEADERSHIP, MERGERS, AND LOCATIONS

A stellar group of dental faculty, a series of mergers with other schools, and three different locations for the school characterized the years after the establishment of the dental school at Columbia University.

Leadership

Between 1916 and 1927, the Columbia University Dental School was led by an administrative board that included the dean of the medical school, Samuel Lambert, and after 1919, his successor William Darrach. Also on the board were William J. Gies and two leading New York City dentists, Henry S. Dunning and Henry W. Gillett. Nicholas Murray Butler, the Columbia University president, was closely involved with the development of the dental school and believed that medical and dental students should receive comparable education. James Chidester Egbert, PhD, head of the University's Extension Department, served as chair of the administrative board until Frank Thorn Van Woert took over in 1920 as professor and chair of the administrative board. Van Woert was a leader in the use of X rays in dentistry and an inventor of color photography in oral surgery. Van Woert was born in the town of Halfmoon in Saratoga County, New York, but his family moved to Brooklyn when he was a small boy. He left home when he was twelve years old and worked as an apprentice in a sewing machine factory in Newark, New Jersey.

Van Woert studied dentistry with two dentists and registered as a dentist under an 1879 law that permitted the practice of dentistry after successful completion of the Regents Exams. He was awarded a master of dental science by the New York State Board in 1890 and served as professor of dental surgery and electro-therapeutics for six years at the University of Buffalo. Van Woert was the first dentist to lead the school, and he was called the director, not the dean. Actually, Van Woert was a member of the school's administrative board, which ran the school. He became chair of the board in 1920. The 1928 yearbook was dedicated to his memory. It noted, in addition to his other accomplishments, that he worked to bring dental care to children in the public schools of New York City. It also noted that although he was not successful in that endeavor, it was not because of his tireless efforts.

Van Woert was one of a group of outstanding individuals who led the dental school in its early years. Two leading dentists of the day, William and Henry Dunning, were founding members of the school. Henry Dunning held the dual degrees of DMD (New York College of

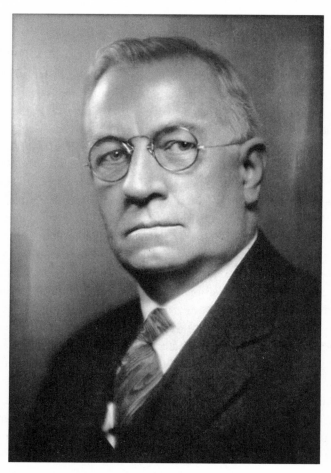

FIGURE 1.2 Dr. Frank Thorn Van Woert was named the director of the Columbia University Dental School in 1920 but was in a leadership position at the school during its earliest years.

Dentistry 1904) and MD (College of Physicians and Surgeons 1911) and was an oral surgeon who sailed on the Saint Louis in 1917 with the Presbyterian Hospital unit to serve during World War I. Henry's brother William was an early proponent of the treatment of periodontal disease. The Dunning brothers' grandfather was also a dentist in New York City. William Dunning's son, James Dunning, was a 1930 graduate of the School of Dental and Oral Surgery, and in 1947 at the age of thirty-five became dean of the Harvard School of Dental Medicine.

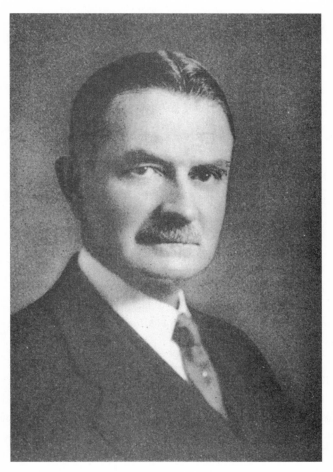

FIGURE 1.3 Dr. William Bailey Dunning, a prominent dental practitioner in New York City, worked closely with William J. Gies to prepare the school's founding document. He served on the faculty in the periodontic department.

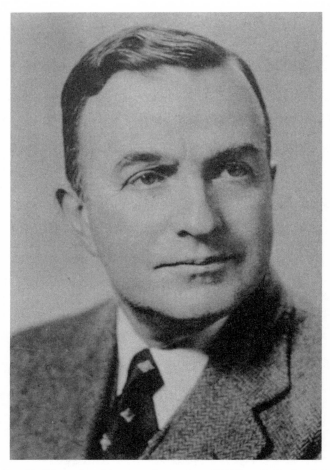

FIGURE 1.4 Dr. Henry Sage Dunning, the brother of William Bailey, headed the Department of Oral Surgery in the school and held an appointment in the Presbyterian Hospital.

William Dunning and William Gies were close colleagues throughout the founding of the dental school and during the time Gies was preparing his report for the Carnegie Foundation. In fact, according to William J. Gies II, the grandson of the Columbia founder, Gies worked on the report most nights and often into the early morning hours. His grandson also recalled that Gies would call William Dunning on the telephone late in the night, which disturbed the Dunning household. Dunning may also have had a hand in writing the 1916 founding document, *A Dental School on University Lines* (see Appendix 1 for the founding document). The founding document is not attributed to one author, but most believe that William Gies and William Dunning drafted it together. The vision for the dental school presented in the founding document recognized the importance of a high-quality dental education in collaboration with the medical school at Columbia and set the stage for the College of Dental Medicine, as these brief excerpts attest:

(1) "Dentistry and Dental Education are on the threshold of extraordinary development but are unable to take advantage of their opportunities because of the traditional separation of dentistry and medicine."

(2) " . . . Leading dentists and physicians of New York . . . proposed to connect the new school of dentistry with the proposed new medical centre, to be established by Columbia University and the Presbyterian Hospital . . ."

(3) "It is proposed to make the dental course at Columbia one of four years, the first two years of which are to be identical with, and part of, the medical course."

(4) "A dental dispensary . . . as a basis for scientific research will be one of the large features of the new school."

(5) "With the first two years of a medical course as a foundation, the increased clinical material, bedside instruction in hospital wards and the greatly enlarged laboratory facilities which the new school will provide will all make for better and more scientifically trained dentists."

This vision of dentistry and dental education was forward thinking, especially since dentistry had not previously been considered important enough to include in medical education. It recognized that the two fields' schools should be connected through colocation and through a combined curriculum in the first two years of professional education. Many of the themes in the founding document were carried over by Gies into his 1926 report to the Carnegie Foundation.

Those leading dentists who were listed members of the founding document—William J. Gies, Henry Dunning, William Dunning, Henry Gillett, Leuman Waugh, and William Jarvie—played major roles in translating this vision into the Columbia University Dental School over the next two to three decades. In fact, Henry Dunning was an oral surgeon who served as head of dentistry at the old Vanderbilt Clinic located at Sixtieth Street and Tenth Avenue. This connection to the Vanderbilt Clinic would serve the dental school well later on when the Vanderbilt Clinic relocated to 168th Street on the new Columbia–Presbyterian Medical Center campus. Henry Dunning also played a major role in fund-raising for the dental school. These early leaders were required to raise the funds necessary to launch the dental school. From 1921 through 1929, gifts to the school totaled $311,973.44 ($4 million in 2014 dollars).

Van Woert served as the director of the school until 1927, when Alfred Owre was appointed as dean of the school. Owre would prove to be a controversial choice. Alfred Owre was one of the leading dental educators in the country. He held both the DMD and MD degrees. He was born in Norway during his family's trip to their homeland for a Christmas visit. Subsequently, the family returned home to Minneapolis

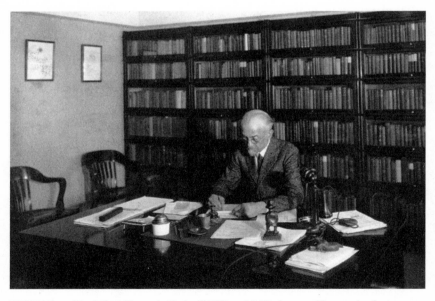

FIGURE 1.5 Dr. Alfred Owre held the DMD and MD degrees. He was the first person to hold the title of dean and joined the dental school in 1927.

SCULPTORS LIPTON AND FERBER AND THE "DELICATE PROFESSION" OF DENTISTRY

Dean Alfred Owre was a proponent of a broad liberal education for dentists. He wrote that "the whole world of artistic endeavor—literature, music, design, painting, sculpture—every division of the industrial and liberal arts—teems with lessons for the worker in so exacting and delicate a profession as that of dentistry."[8] His understanding of the nature of those who enter the profession was accurate in regard to two graduates of the school—Seymour Lipton and Herbert Ferber Silvers. Born only three years apart (Lipton in 1903 and Ferber in 1906), they graduated in 1927 and 1930, respectively. Both became noted sculptors while maintaining their careers in dentistry. Lipton became well known for his modern abstract expressionist sculptures, one of which, *Winter Solstice #2*, is in the Hirshhorn Museum in Washington, D.C. Herbert Ferber, known as Dr. Herbert Silvers in the dental world, was also an abstract expressionist sculptor. His works are represented in many museums, including the Museum of Modern Art, the Whitney Museum, and

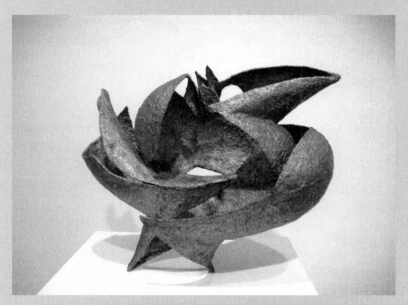

FIGURE 1.6 *Winter Solstice #2* (1957) was created by Seymour Lipton, a 1927 DDS graduate from SDOS. Dr. Lipton was an early modern abstract expressionist sculptor. This work is held in the Hirshhorn Museum in Washington, D.C.

the Guggenheim Museum. In 1973 a large abstract black Cor-Ten steel Ferber sculpture was placed in the front east court of the American Dental Association building in Chicago. In 1992 the sculpture was donated by the American Dental Association to the city of Chicago because a renovation to the front of the building could no longer accommodate the sculpture.

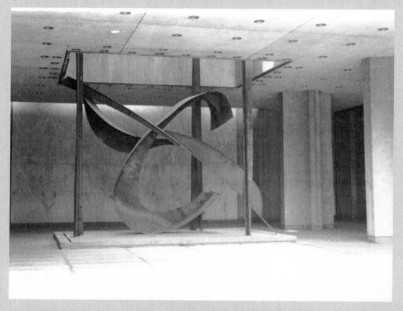

FIGURE 1.7 *Untitled* (1973) was the work of Herbert Ferber, who graduated from SDOS in 1930. He used the name Herbert Ferber in the art world and Dr. Herbert Silvers in the dental world. This sculpture was commissioned by the American Dental Association and placed in front of the ADA headquarters. In 1992 the ADA donated the sculpture to the City of Chicago.

with their son. Owre continued his education in Minnesota; in 1894 he earned his dental degree from the University of Minnesota and then a degree in medicine in 1895. He was appointed dean of the University of Minnesota dental school in 1905 at the age of thirty-four.

Alfred Owre was also a man who loved to walk. His biographer estimated that during his lifetime he walked 120,000 miles. His treks

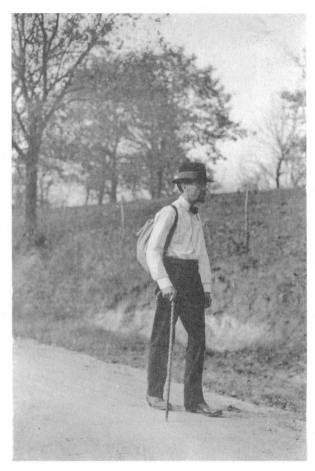

FIGURE 1.8 Dr. Alfred Owre was dean from 1927 to 1934. He is shown here on one of his many treks. It is estimated he walked more than 120,000 miles during his lifetime; this included a hike from Chicago to New York City. (Photo courtesy of University of Minnesota Archives, University of Minnesota-Twin Cities.)

included trips across Russia, China, and Japan and a hike from Chicago to New York in 1924. He usually walked 25 miles each day. He was over six feet tall and weighed only 125 pounds.

This very unusual man was well known in dental circles even before he came to Columbia as dean in 1927. He was very familiar with the ideal dental school that Columbia University was creating in New York. He admired the fact that the dental and medical schools were closely connected. Prior to his appointment as dean of the Columbia University Dental School, Owre was dean at the University of Minnesota Dental School, and he strengthened the Columbia faculty by bringing in seventeen professors from Minnesota.

Owre's deanship, however, became a tortuous period both for him personally and for the Columbia University Dental School. His deanship lasted until 1933, and it best can be described as "stormy." Some of this was fueled by his relationship with William Gies. As a leader in the founding of the dental school, Gies admired Owre and consulted with him during the Carnegie study. There was no doubt that Owre was a leading intellectual and subscribed to the school's founding document. However, he and Gies parted ways after the publication of the Gies report, which did not mesh well with the new dean's thoughts.

Like Gies, Owre was a vocal proponent of closing what were known as the "commercial for-profit" dental schools in favor of university-based schools. And while he firmly believed that dental schools should be part of the university system in the United States, as did Gies, differences arose over Owre's belief that dentistry should develop as an integral part of medicine. Conversely, Gies indicated in the report that it should remain a separate profession for practical reasons. Both were passionate about their views on dentistry in relation to medicine. Owre was both a physician and dentist, and he believed that dentistry should be integrated within medicine, not separated from it. Owre's true intention regarding what should happen to dental schools was revealed in a letter to President Butler in 1932; he wrote, "As you know, I have long believed that the desirable and logical end for all dental schools were for them to become departments of reputable medical schools. The biological unit of the human body, alone, makes this a logical development . . . I feel that we should ultimately cease to give the D.D.S. degree, unless other special degrees be given in other departments of the medical school . . . At Columbia, we have made a beginning."[9] Most likely, Gies knew Owre's private thoughts on this critical matter. But he also realized that because the two fields had "grown up" separately and had separate organizations, the traditions that had evolved could not be broken to bring dentistry into medicine. So he took the practical route: dentistry was to be closely aligned with but not part of medicine. This did not sit well with Owre, and the once close colleagues now became estranged because of their differing visions for their profession.

Owre's relationship with the dental society in New York was also problematic. This was due to his ideas on how the profession should emerge and because he had proposed a "fee" clinic rather than a charity clinic in what would become the new Vanderbilt Clinic facility on 168th Street. He said that there was the need for a "place where discriminating people of moderate means can go and get dependable service . . . [at] the service clinic in connection with a high grade teaching institution."[10] By this he meant the new clinic in Washington Heights, into which he would move the school in September 1928, would charge fees, and attract many middle-class patients. He estimated there would be about 40,000 to 50,000 such patients.

The dentists in New York believed that the school would be in competition with their private practices and resisted this new clinic strenuously. A broad thinker, Owre also clashed with the dental establishment for another serious reason: what they termed his elitist attitude toward the profession. He conceived of the dentist as a diagnostician practicing a higher order of treatment. Consequently, he supported the idea that "dental mechanics" should be taught to do the more manual work, while the dentist would be the diagnostician and treat the complex cases. While his vision for the use of dental mechanics never was adopted by the profession and was vigorously opposed, his idea is gaining traction today, some eighty-plus years later, especially with the public, because there are few dentists and great need. A dental therapist who performs some of the basic dental procedures, including using a drill to remove decay, place restorations, and perform simple extractions and prevention procedures, is emerging as a viable extension to the dentist. Again, this type of worker is controversial within the profession. However, several states have passed legislation to permit the practice of dental therapy. Owre was certainly ahead of his time!

The tensions that developed over many of Owre's educational and professional beliefs, as well as his ideas that challenged the practicing community, became so great that the faculty asked President Butler to remove Owre as dean. In 1933 Butler provided Owre with a leave of absence and appointed Willard Rappleye, dean of the medical school, to serve in the dual capacity of dean of the medical school and acting dean of the dental school. The trustees accepted Owre's resignation in 1934, and he died in 1935. There is a building on the University of Minnesota campus named for Owre. An interesting paper by David Nash describes much of the conflict between Owre and Gies.[11]

Despite all the controversy during the period of 1928 to 1933, the dental school continued to make progress. During the first three decades of its existence, the school attracted a talented faculty who accomplished much in the field of research and treatment. For example, Leuman Waugh (1877–1972), one of the early faculty members, became famous for his studies in Alaska. He found that Alaskan Natives' health was adversely affected by the introduction of nontraditional foods. He noted that the Eskimos of Labrador and Alaska were free from caries on native diets consisting of proteins and fats and no fermentable carbohydrate, but when they switched to a diet rich in carbohydrates they had rampant caries. Waugh's photographs of Alaska and its people are in the Smithsonian Collection.

Among others were leaders in the field of periodontology. Periodontal disease was sorely neglected at the time and the knowledge base of the causes and treatment, other than scaling and oral hygiene, was lacking. William Dunning, Isador Hirschfeld, and Harold Leonard, all faculty in the early years of the dental school, and later Frank Beube and Robert Gottsegen, along with many others on the faculty over the century, made Columbia the mecca of periodontology.

Arthur T. Rowe (1883–1935) joined the Columbia University Dental School faculty in 1927. He was born in North Dakota and practiced in Larimore in that same state. He was well respected in the town and became its mayor. He moved to Minneapolis in 1917 and eventually joined the faculty at the University prior to coming to New York. Rowe was chair of prosthodontics at Columbia, an important field because so many people had their teeth extracted due to dental caries that replacing them with prosthetic appliances became an important course in dental schools. The students dedicated the 1931 yearbook to Dr. Rowe, calling him an individual they all looked up to as a teacher and a man. Sadly, Rowe became the victim of a terrible crime (which we will revisit later in the chapter) that represented a turning point in the dental school.

Mergers

During this same time period, the dental school merged with a post-graduate school, a dental hygiene school, and the College of Dental and Oral Surgery.

In 1917, shortly after the Columbia University Board of Trustees approved the dental school to admit students, the New York Post-graduate School of Dentistry and the New York School of Dental Hygiene were both absorbed by the University and administered by the University Extension Department. Eventually, both became integrated into the dental school and administered by it rather than by the University Extension.

The New York Post-graduate School of Dentistry was located at 35 West Thirty-Ninth Street. Frank Van Woert, the chair of its administrative staff, was to become the first director of the Columbia University Dental School. Henry Gillett (DMD, Harvard 1885) was the leader behind the New York Post-graduate School. Leading dentists in New York urged the board of directors of the Post-graduate School to merge the school with Columbia so that it would be under the umbrella of a university. On May 11, 1917, the postgraduate school was transferred to Columbia. A flyer announced that Columbia University offered advanced courses in dentistry. One of them, offered by Dr. John Oppie McCall, was Symptomatology of Perodontoclasia: Cardinal Symptoms. Oppie McCall was one of the early leaders in the field of periodontics. Gillett joined the faculty of the dental school as a professor and served on the faculty into the 1940s. He was a well-respected member of the faculty and the class of 1934 dedicated its yearbook to him, calling him a wise and inspiring faculty member. Columbia attracted interest in postdoctoral education from its inception because of the merger with the New York Post-graduate School. This continues today. In this, William J. Gies was again prescient. He had recognized the need for a period of postgraduate study after graduation from dental school and recommended that postgraduate studies become widely available for graduates.

The dental hygiene school functioned as part of the School of Dental and Oral Surgery for sixty-five years, from 1917 until 1982, when the courses in dental hygiene were terminated. A section later in this chapter describes the early years of the merger of the dental hygiene school into the university and the dental school, and Chapter 3 will describe the circumstances of the closure of the program, which educated the leadership for the early formation of dental hygiene programs in the United States.

In 1923 the Columbia University Dental School then merged again with the larger College of Dental and Oral Surgery (CDOS) of New York, a non-university-affiliated proprietary dental school located in two buildings on East Thirty-Fourth and Thirty-Fifth Streets. Originally called the New York College of Dental Surgery, the school was founded in 1852 in Syracuse, New York. It was the first dental college in New York State and the fifth to be established in the United States. Dr. Amos Westcott, a leading citizen in Syracuse and an influential dentist of the time, was the founder. Westcott earned his MD from the Albany Medical College in 1840 and studied dentistry while in medical school. He devoted his career to dentistry rather than medicine and was awarded an honorary DDS degree from the Baltimore College of Dental Surgery in 1843. Interestingly, Westcott trained Edwin James Dunning, the grandfather of SDOS founders Drs. William B. and Henry Sage Dunning and the great-grandfather of James Dunning (DDS, SDOS 1930), a future dean of the Harvard School of Dental Medicine. The Syracuse school was located at 6 Salinas Street, but shortly after it became operational, it was destroyed by a fire in 1856. Subsequently, the school's charter was moved to New York City and was incorporated into the New York College of Dental and Oral Surgery charter some years later in 1892. Appendix 2 provides more information about the predecessor institutions and their relationship to the formation of the School of Dental and Oral Surgery.

William Carr, MD, DDS, led the College of Dental and Oral Surgery. It was established as a freestanding school unaffiliated with a university. By 1922, however, the College of Dental and Oral Surgery was found deficient by the Dental Educational Council. The council urged the school to merge with a university. The College of Dental and Oral Surgery was taken over by Columbia University and merged with the Columbia University Dental School in 1923.

Locations

The dental school started carrying out the terms of its founding document in 1916 in space in the medical school building on Fifty-Ninth Street.

The University located the dental school with the then well-established Columbia University Medical School, close to Roosevelt Hospital. In 1920 a small four-story building was constructed next to the medical school for the dental school. It housed modern dental chairs, electric engines, fountain cuspidors, and the students' private cabinets. Research labs were on the third floor of the building. However, the school did not remain there long, as the series of previously described mergers affected its location.

Just seven years later, in 1923, the dental school moved again, after merging with the College of Dental and Oral Surgery. Through the merger, the school inherited two buildings on East Thirty-Fourth and Thirty-Fifth Streets. However, it did not remain there for long.

The plans for the dental school to move to the new medical school building on 168th Street were already in place when the University took possession of the Thirty-Fourth and Thirty-Fifth Street buildings, which at that time were valued at more than $400,000 to $500,000 ($5.4 to $6.5 million in 2014 dollars). The facilities of the College of Dental and

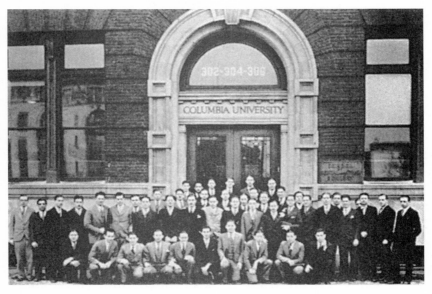

FIGURE 1.9 The Columbia University Dental School moved from its first location on Fifty-Ninth Street adjacent to the College of Physicians and Surgeons building into the two buildings owned by the College of Dental and Oral Surgery on East Thirty-Fourth and Thirty-Fifth Streets shown in this photograph from the 1920s.

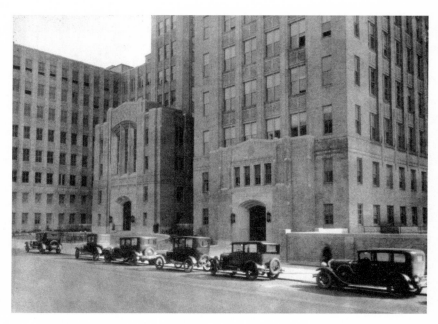

FIGURE 1.10 Shown here are the entrances to the College of Physicians and Surgeons and Vanderbilt Clinic buildings on West 168th Street. In 1928 the dental school, now known as the School of Dental and Oral Surgery, moved from East Thirty-Fourth and Thirty-Fifth Streets into three floors of the Vanderbilt Clinic building (the left entrance) of the Presbyterian Hospital.

Oral Surgery on Thirty-Fourth and Thirty-Fifth Streets were eight miles away from where the medical school would be located in Washington Heights. The distance made it impossible for students in the dental school to attend classes with the medical students. So, in 1928 the dental school followed the medical school to the Washington Heights location on West 168th Street upon completion of the construction of the medical campus there. The top three stories of the new Vanderbilt Clinic were built for the dental school—a smaller facility, but a greater opportunity.

The Significance of the Merger of the Columbia University Dental School with the College of Dental and Oral Surgery

Until the merger with the College of Dental and Oral Surgery, the Columbia University Dental School had a very small enrollment, partly due to its

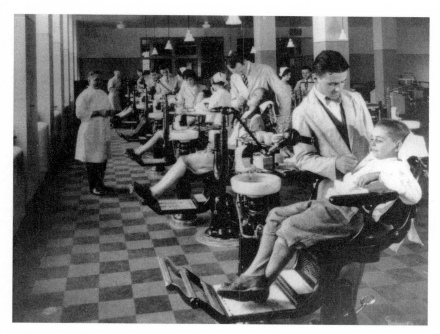

FIGURE 1.11 The pediatric dentistry clinic (shown ca. 1932) in the Vanderbilt Clinic building was a busy service in early times and still is today, although in a different location. Dr. Ewing McBeath, who held both the MD and DDS degrees, supervises the care provided by dental and dental hygiene students.

high admissions standards and partly due to the effects of World War I. The first two students entering the Columbia University Dental School were Joseph Schroff and Sidney Kramer. They graduated with both DDS (1920) and MD (1922) degrees after completing a six-year combined program. Joseph Schroff joined the dental school faculty and the attending staff of Presbyterian Hospital. By 1923 the student body had a total of nineteen students. Prior to 1920, only four students were enrolled each year, growing to a student body of twenty in the 1922–1923 year, just before the merger. However, with the merger, Columbia absorbed all the enrolled students in the proprietary College of Dental and Oral Surgery. In 1923, 547 students matriculated; 32 were women and 171 graduated. After the merger, the class size was reduced to about ninety students per class and further reduced with the move to the new but smaller site in Washington Heights. In 1928 only thirty-five students graduated.

The merger with the larger independent College of Dental and Oral Surgery was a definite benefit to the development of the Columbia University Dental School. The former was an ongoing school for more than twenty years with 68,000 square feet of buildings and facilities, faculty, and an extensive patient care service. For example, in the year of the merger, 1923–1924, the College of Dental and Oral Surgery provided 66,906 patient visits. In contrast, Columbia's dental school occupied only a small four-story building, an annex to the medical school. However, the College of Dental and Oral Surgery had major academic deficiencies and, while the Columbia University Dental School was the smaller of the two, the higher academic standards of Columbia University prevailed in the merger. The name of the Columbia University Dental School changed, as part of the agreement, to the School of Dental and Oral Surgery (SDOS), a name used until 2006, when it was changed to the College of Dental Medicine.

The dean of the College of Dental and Oral Surgery at the time of the merger, William Carr, MD, DDS, became honorary director (dean) of the merged school. Carr was a respected oral surgeon. He served as president of the American Dental Association from 1907 to 1908.

The merger with the larger College of Dental and Oral Surgery worked well, even though there were major differences in the student body between the original Columbia University Dental School and the newly integrated College of Dental and Oral Surgery. The students enrolled in the Columbia University Dental School were required to enter with two years of college. This requirement, established in 1919, made Columbia the first dental school with such a mandate. The students who entered the College of Dental and Oral Surgery, however, had no such prerequisite and only had to complete high school. In spite of the lack of prerequisite college work, the enrolled students were able to measure up to the Columbia University Dental School standards. Most likely, they were able to meet the higher Columbia University standards because the faculty of the College of Dental and Oral Surgery was embellished with the faculty of the Columbia University Dental School.

The student editors of the 1928 yearbook noted this about the new educational merger in the foreword: "We are now at the close of the first four-year period since Columbia University adopted the College of Dental and Oral Surgery. The first class to have completed four full years of instruction under the University's supervision is about to leave us. With these thoughts in mind, the idea of this volume became a reality. Its purpose is to set a precedent for all years, to unite all classes in the Spirit of our Alma Mater."[12] The transition now complete, the class size was reduced, and in 1928, 1929, and 1930 the classes had thirty-three students, while the class of 1931 grew to sixty-six students. The merger with the College of Dental and Oral Surgery appeared to give the Columbia University Dental School, now the School of Dental and Oral Surgery, "a shot in the arm," as it then began to enroll a sufficient cadre of well-qualified students, many of whom eventually became faculty.

The Course of Study: 1917–1941

During this period the dental curriculum evolved and was reshaped. The course of study outlined in the University's first bulletin or announcement in 1917 was a five-year program. True to its original document, the first two years were identical to the courses taken by the medical students. In the first year, however, in addition to the basic science courses, dental students took two courses in dentistry: operative dentistry and prosthodontia. In the second year, in addition to the basic sciences, dental students took the practice of medicine course, clinics, and predental courses. The third year consisted entirely of dental courses with laboratory and lectures but no clinics. The fourth and fifth years included lectures and clinics.

By 1921, the program changed to four years in length and involved thirty-one school weeks. But again in 1929 the length of the program changed; the school offered a three-year curriculum of forty-four school weeks each year. Most likely, Owre, the dean at that time, was influenced by the Gies report's recommendation that the dental school curriculum be three years in length with students taking postgraduate studies afterward. Actually, Gies had recommended in his report a two-three graduate plan: two years of college prerequisites, three years of dental school, and one or more years of postgraduate training. But the faculty at Columbia did not support the three-year plan for the dental curriculum. In a letter to Van Woert from Henry Gillett, Gillett indicated that Gies was "very sore that Columbia does not endorse the two-three-graduate plan for which I suspect he blames me [Gillett] in particular."[13]

By 1932 Alfred Owre returned the school to the four-year, thirty-one-week curriculum because he said it was difficult to secure teachers in the summertime and the strain on the students during the hot New York summers was too great. Under Owre's leadership, the curriculum offered 140 hours of electives, which could be selected in the basic sciences and in thirteen clinical areas. Students also took a course in psychiatry and in public health, which included preventive medicine and public health administration. Each senior in 1941 was required to present a thesis representing original reading, scientific research, or both. The seniors were also required to take a comprehensive examination toward the end of their academic year.

By 1920, the dental school was offering advanced courses in dentistry for practitioners at the 437 West Fifty-Ninth Street location. Courses covered the following subjects: oral diagnosis including radiology, oral surgery, anesthesia, exodontia, plate prosthesis, dental ceramics, cast gold inlay, root canal technique, periodontia, and removable bridgework. In 1929–1930 graduate courses were offered that led to the master of arts or doctor of philosophy degrees. Through the University's Extension Division, practitioners could arrange advanced studies with each of the dental school's divisions. These divisions could accommodate two or three dentists for advanced study in the clinical practice of dentistry.

In 1927 the school offered a twelve-month course for graduates to prepare them for specialization in orthodontia. The bulletin of that year indicated that there were 600 patients under orthodontic treatment "affording unsurpassed opportunity for gaining a broad clinical experience." Three students were assigned to a teacher. Didactic instruction included weekly conferences, special lectures on biology, embryology and histology, anatomy, child psychology, facial art, photography, and metallurgy. A certificate of proficiency in orthodontia was awarded at the end of the twelve-month period and "upon those whose qualifications are acceptable to the Graduate Faculties of Columbia University, the Master's degree may be conferred for work completed in this department."[14] In addition, by the 1939–1940 academic year it was possible for the graduates to take a one-year course leading to the degree of master of science in public health. There was clearly recognition that dentistry required specialists in certain areas of practice that involved advanced education for dentists to gain broader knowledge in public health.

The total cost of attending the dental school in its opening year in 1916–1917 averaged $828 ($15,054 in 2014 dollars), of which $240 ($4,363 in 2014 dollars) was for tuition. By the 1928–1929 year, the total cost had almost doubled, rising to $1,566 ($21,452 in 2014 dollars), of which $460 ($6,301 in 2014 dollars) was for tuition. The rise in cost of education seems to have been a factor in dental education then as it is today.

Two Murders and a Suicide: Moving On

In addition to the tumultuous mergers and location changes, in 1935 the dental school was shaken by the tragic murder of the associate dean and a faculty member, the shooting of another professor, and the suicide of the murderer.

By the 1934–1935 year, following the resignation of Alfred Owre, the school was administered by committees under the leadership of Dean Willard Rappleye, the dean of the medical school. The committees were the administration, curriculum, library, extension and postgraduate courses, and the research committees. Arthur Rowe provided the day-to-day leadership as associate dean. Having grown up in Casselton, North Dakota, he received his DDS in 1906 at the University of Minnesota. He was one of the faculty members brought in earlier by Alfred Owre. Rowe served as head of the Division of Prosthodontics after arriving at Columbia in 1926.

One December day in 1935, Arthur Rowe was sitting at his desk when a handyman in the school shot and killed him. Then, the handyman ran through the school and murdered faculty member Dr. Paul Wiberg as well. When Dr. William Crawford came to the aid of Dr. Wiberg, he was also shot, but not fatally. The *Columbia Spectator* headline on December 13, 1935, was "3 Professors Shot at Medical Center by Crazed Technician; Rowe, Wiberg Dead, Crawford Wounded; Assassin Suicide." A letter to Arthur Rowe from the murderer, dated October 28, 1935, was found on Rowe's desk. The letter accused Rowe of being unjust and prejudiced against the murderer and threatened Rowe (see Appendix 3 for the text of the letter).

The story went on to report that the assassin was Victor Koussow, once an officer in the Russian army, now a laboratory technician at the dental school. Rowe had fired Koussow shortly after Koussow quarreled

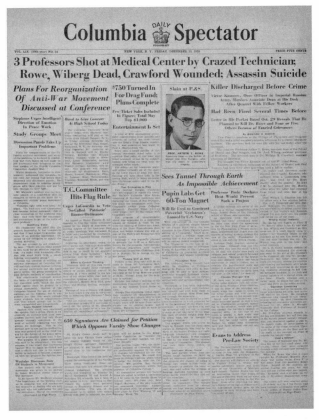

FIGURE 1.12 This headline in the December 13, 1935, edition of the *Columbia Spectator* says it all: the tragic murder of the associate dean Arthur Rowe and faculty member Paul Wiberg while faculty member William Crawford was wounded. The two murders and shooting of Crawford shocked the university community.

with a coworker. Koussow was described in the article as an individual with a persecution complex. The article described the following events: "The killer went racing down the corridor waving his revolver and chasing the mechanic with whom he had been quarreling in the morning, evidently intending to kill him. He menaced students in the hall and scared patients at a dental clinic on the floor. Finally, running into a locker room, he placed the gun to his heart, fired and killed himself as the police arrived."[15]

ALUMNI VOICES: NATHAN (NAT) SHECKMAN—A STUDENT REMEMBERS THE SHOOTING OF 1935

The aftermath of the killing of Arthur Rowe and Paul Wiberg and the wounding of William Crawford "sent shock waves through the student body" according to Nathan (Nat) Sheckman, class of 1938. Sheckman, a freshman student at the time, was in a medical school class in microbiology when the chaos erupted. He recalls, "My classmates and I looked out of the windows and saw the bodies of those killed being wheeled out of the building!"

His recollection of that day and his time at SDOS permits a look back at the school as it was eighty-one years ago. In a telephone interview,[16] he shared reflections on his time at the school. His father, Herman Sheckman, graduated in 1909 from the College of Dental and Oral Surgery of New York, the school Columbia incorporated into the School of Dental and Oral Surgery in 1923. He spoke warmly of the faculty; for example, he cited Carl Oman, a professor of operative dentistry, as a "wonderful man who was empathetic to students and a great man." He spoke fondly of Henry Gillett as a role model for "how to conduct yourself and behave as a professional person."

Sheckman enjoyed his time at SDOS. He was fortunate because his family lived in an apartment at 23 Haven Avenue, now the site of one of the Columbia towers on Haven Avenue. This allowed him close access to the medical center and the library, in which he spent many hours studying. He recalled that two weeks before his finals in senior year, he came down with mononucleosis and was too sick to take his exams. The then associate dean, Houghton Holiday, exempted him from his finals, which was a great relief. He also learned by mail a few days later that he had been elected to OKU, the honorary dental society that accepts only the top 10 percent of the class as new members. The 1938 yearbook called Sheckman "a man who has the best qualities of gentlemanliness" and "one of the finest of the fine." He served as class president for three years and was a member of the William Jarvie Society. Nat met his wife Ruth (now deceased) while in dental school.

They married soon after graduation, had two sons, and celebrated their seventy-third anniversary in May of 2012. Before retiring to Florida, Nat had a forty-year practice of dentistry, first in an office in Parkchester, New York, and then in the New York Central Building on Park Avenue. He was the director of a preventive service for the Seagram's Company and served as the president of the alumni organization in 1967–1968.

The students dedicated the 1936 yearbook to both Arthur Rowe and Paul Wiberg. Rowe was only forty-seven years old when he was killed. The students described him as an individual with a sense of humor, friendliness, and ample common sense that rendered the complicated into the simple. Paul Wiberg was also a Minnesotan who received his DDS in 1920. In the yearbook, the students lauded Wiberg's use of motion pictures to demonstrate the construction of crowns and bridges and his scientific approach to the treatment of bite closure cases. He was only thirty-eight years old when he was killed and was a promising young faculty member. These sad events weighed heavily on the school. The students, in remembering the tragedy, wrote in the yearbook that the "needless loss of these valuable lives brings not only grief and deprivation to their families, but a sense of personal bereavement to every member of our organization whether of the faculty, student body or staff."

There is an interesting fact about the murderer, Victor Koussow. Upon his emigration to the United States from Russia, his behavior caused him to be assessed by what was then called the lunacy commission. Mayor Fiorello LaGuardia was a member of that commission. The commission examined Koussow three times after hearing the testimony of Dr. Perry Lichtenstein, who evaluated Koussow in the following way: "He is a psychopathic and erratic man and may some day develop insanity; but at the present there is no indication."[17] It is too bad the commission did not bar him entrance to the country!

After the tragic events, Dr. Houghton Holiday took over as associate dean and served until the 1945–1946 academic year. According to the 1937 *Dental Columbian* yearbook, the students believed that Dr. Holiday was the right person to step in after the tragic events of 1935 and heal the wounds of the school. Holiday was yet another faculty member brought in from the University of Minnesota (where he had received his DDS degree in 1917) and was a professor of radiology.

Holiday was a forward-looking educator who reflected on the development of the profession during the first three decades of the twentieth century. He was aware that times were changing. "There are changing and growing demands being made upon the profession which must be reflected in the teaching program . . . It is very easy to be tied down to the past, accepting what is, as what should be.

We need to tear ourselves loose from tradition and periodically, if not constantly, readjust our profession to the changes which are taking place."[18] His statement about the need for readjusting dentistry to changes taking place proved prophetic for the twenty-first century as once again we find ourselves in changing times.

Dental Hygiene Becomes Integrated into Columbia University and the Dental School

At about the same time that the dental school at Columbia was established, the field of dental hygiene was developing. Alfred Fones (DDS, New York College of Dentistry 1891) is credited with establishing the field of dental hygiene. As the director of the Dental Division of the Department of Public Health in Bridgeport, Connecticut, he started the first training program for dental hygienists. He had convinced the State of Connecticut that dental hygienists placed in the school system could dramatically improve the oral health of children. As evidence of the efficacy of prevention in dental care, he presented the results of the five-year pilot program he conducted in the school system. Over a five-year period, children who had received teeth cleanings and oral hygiene instructions from dental hygienists had 33.9 to 49.6 percent less caries in their permanent teeth. This demonstrated the importance of a preventive approach to the treatment of dental caries, which were then rampant in schoolchildren.

Also around this time, the New York School of Dental Hygiene was established as part of the old Vanderbilt Clinic. Dr. Louise Ball, DDS, a faculty member at Hunter College, was the founding director of the school. Dr. Ball was an early proponent of providing preventive dental services for New York City schoolchildren. She even devised a way to pay for those services by suggesting schoolchildren should pay 1 cent per week for preventive dental services and have a school stamp book to show they had paid their 1 cent. She calculated that would generate $10,000 per week from the 1 million New York City schoolchildren.

Women who were at least nineteen years of age and had completed at least one year of high school were admitted to the New York School of Dental Hygiene. After taking summer courses at Hunter, students attended Vanderbilt Clinic for the remainder of the one-year program.

Alfred Fones was a faculty member at Columbia and, with Louise Ball, helped the merger of the fledgling Dental Hygiene School in New York City with the Columbia University Dental School. On May 2, 1917, the transfer of the Dental Hygiene School to Columbia was effected. The highly experienced Dr. Louise Ball became the director of the program. The program was offered through Columbia's Department of University Extension and was listed in the annual bulletin of the dental school under the title "Courses in Dental Hygiene." It was the first dental hygiene program in a university, and the second dental hygiene school in the country. Similar programs were established at the Forsyth Dental Infirmary for Children and at the Rochester Dental Dispensary. The total number of dental hygiene graduates at Columbia over the first ten years (1917 through 1926) was 423, with a low of seven in 1920 and a high of ninety-three in 1917 (the average number of graduates, excluding the high and the low, was forty graduates per year).

By the 1920–1921 year, the admissions requirements at Columbia for the courses in dental hygiene included four years of high school. By the following year, the program was placed under the administrative board of the dental school rather than the University's Extension Department. Professor of Preventive Dentistry Anna Hughes, who received her DMD from Tufts in 1909, was in charge of the program. Interestingly, Dr. Fones also taught courses in preventive dentistry and oral hygiene to the second-, third-, and fourth-year dental students in 1920. The dental student courses included practice in removing deposits and stains through a systematic technique of instrumentation that progressed from manikins to patients.

By the 1926–1927 year, the school's bulletin stated that the courses in dental hygiene were offered by the School of Dental and Oral Surgery, and that Professor Hughes, instead of Dr. Fones, was presenting the course in preventive dentistry to the dental students. Dr. Hughes remained in charge of the dental hygiene program through this period of time and was joined by two dental hygienist instructors, Katherine Hollis and Geneva Walls. Dr. Hughes noted in the 1933 *Dental Columbian* yearbook that a number of graduates wanted education in teaching, and so they continued at the State Teachers College of Buffalo, where postgraduate training was offered. There they could earn a certificate as dental hygiene teachers. In the same year, there were fifty graduates from the dental hygiene program.

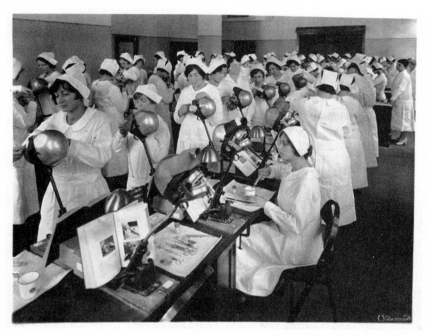

FIGURE 1.13 In 1917 the newly formed New York School of Dental Hygiene was absorbed into the Columbia University Dental School as courses in dental hygiene. Dr. Anna Hughes (DMD, Tufts 1909), the director, can be seen on the far right supervising a preclinical techniques class (ca. 1928).

Achieving Its Standards

As we have seen, the period from the founding of the school in 1916 to 1941 was a tumultuous and exciting time. Led by a distinguished group of dentists in New York, the University and medical school understood that dentistry was an important component of health care. The University established a school that would uphold its standards in both education and scholarship. Moving the field of dentistry into research, including student research, became one of the tenets of the new school at Columbia. The University president was deeply involved with the school's development, as were the deans of the medical school. William J. Gies became the guiding light for the new school at Columbia, and Alfred Owre, although controversial, brought in a talented group of faculty from the University of Minnesota to augment an already accomplished group of practitioners.

William Gies called for the formation of a student honor society for the promotion of the spirit of research among students in the dental school. He recommended it be named for Jarvie, a member of the founding committee who was interested in dental research and whose brother was a major benefactor of the school. The William Jarvie Society was formed in 1920.

The society helped the school develop according to the high standards that were expected. The *Dental Columbian* yearbook of 1941 included a section on research demonstrating that the school practiced what it preached. There were summaries of twenty-six ongoing investigations in the school, each with a student and faculty sponsor. While all of the summaries are fascinating, two will be mentioned here because they represent intriguing hints of the school's future.

The first, a study entitled "Ovarian Hormone Influence on Keratinization of the Oral Mucosa as Determined by Correlation with the Menstrual Cycle," was carried out by two students, Irving Kittay and Saul Kamen, and sponsored by Dr. Dan Ziskin. Saul Kamen would go on to become a world expert in geriatric dentistry. His son Paul was a 1975 graduate of the dental school. Paul joined the faculty after completing postgraduate training in periodontics at Harvard and serves on the faculty today. Irving Kittay became a faculty member in the treatment of temporomandibular joint disorders. Dan Ziskin became the head of the division of stomatology.

The second study was "A Study of the Effect of Vitamin D on Salivary Calcium and Phosphorus," conducted by students Melvin Morris, Irving Weinberg, and Emanuel Knishkowy. The faculty sponsor was Max Karshan, a colleague of Dr. Gies. Melvin Morris, who would go on to produce a number of well-known studies in periodontal pathology, became a well-respected member of the periodontal faculty and served through the 1980s.

The founding principles, mergers, and location changes continued to strengthen the school. In 1935 the school became fully integrated with the medical school, with the dean of medicine also serving in the dual role as dean of dentistry. Having developed during World War I, the Roaring Twenties, and the Great Depression of the 1930s, the school, like all others in the nation, would soon face World War II. It would strive to keep up the high standards its founders had created for a dental school along university lines—that is, Columbia University lines.

While Gies and Owre may have differed on how dentistry should be positioned in relation to medicine—Gies thought for practical reasons dentistry should be an independent profession, closely aligned with medicine, whereas Owre believed it should be a specialty of medicine—they both agreed that dental schools should be centers of research. In fact, Owre wrote about this in 1929 shortly after arriving at Columbia as dean. In his first annual report he said: "It is the hope of the [Columbia] school to maintain applied science in close association with pure science. The isolated professional school may develop the art of dentistry, but hardly its science."[19]

Landmark Dental Research Studies in the 1930s

Faculty research in the dental school in its early years played a prominent role. Picking up on some of Gies's early research interests in dental caries, there was a major effort to determine the etiology of the disease. Leuman Waugh had already shown how a change to a diet rich in carbohydrate had caused a high caries rate in Alaskan Natives. In the 1930s, with support from the Commonwealth Fund, the Columbia University Dental Caries Research Committee carried out an in-depth study of dental caries. More than twenty faculty members from the basic science departments and the dental school were involved in these studies. Charles Bodecker, who joined the faculty as a professor of dentistry (oral histology and embryology) in the 1920s and was a 1900 graduate of the Buffalo Dental School, served as chair of the research group. The studies investigated two theories of dental caries: environmental factors such as bacteria and fermentation of "food stuff" adhering to the teeth and the physiological influence of tooth decay through saliva and the dental pulp.

This multiyear study was a landmark in many ways. For example, Theodore Rosebury, who joined the faculty in 1932 as an instructor in bacteriology and was a graduate of the University of Pennsylvania Dental School in 1928, succeeded in producing dental caries in an animal model. He was able to show that the rate of decay in animal teeth could be controlled by dietary and environmental regulation.

Bodecker and colleagues did a series of studies on structural elements of enamel with reference to resistance to acid and, with Rosebury, investigated bacterial invasion of the enamel. Rosebury, in collaboration with others, investigated acid-forming bacteria. Bodecker had earlier shown that enamel contained organic content, contrary to the prevailing notion. The research team published more than thirty-eight papers on the outcome of this large-scale dental caries investigation.

Other faculty built on this model. Solomon Rosenstein, a 1930 SDOS graduate and director of pedodontics, was conducting studies on rampant caries in young children in reference to its relation to early feeding habits. Rosenstein wrote the first scholarly article on "night bottle caries," which is now called "early childhood caries," a condition that still affects about 20 percent of children under the age of five.[20] The children's dental clinic, established in 1930, conducted prenatal studies and studies on preventing dental caries. This early collaboration of scientists was widespread among the faculty. For example, in the 1940s, Eli Siegel, an assistant in biochemistry, and Benjamin Tennenbaum, a clinical assistant, collaborated with Paul O. Pedersen of the dental school in Copenhagen to study the chemical composition of saliva of caries-free and active-caries patients. Much of the caries research supported by the Commonwealth Fund was reported in a 105-page monograph published by the Columbia University Press in 1940 and prepared by Moses Diamond, associate professor of oral anatomy and a 1914 graduate of New York University Dental School.

The faculty's research interests were broad. Rosebury conducted classic studies using dark-field microscopy to identify fuso-spirochetal infections in the oral cavity. Later he collaborated with the Chest Service at Bellevue Hospital and found that bacteria from the mouth were found in lung abscesses. Isador Hirschfeld, a 1902 graduate from New York University Dental School, teamed up with Daniel Ziskin (DDS, University of Minnesota 1917), a clinical staff member in the early 1930s, to study oral manifestations in the mouth during pregnancy. Lester Cahn, a New York University graduate of 1917, studied fungal infections in the mouth and showed with special stains that melanoblasts could be found in the gingivae. Frank Beube and Herbert Silvers, both volunteers on the faculty in the 1930s, were studying the insertion of bone salts in areas of bone lost due to cysts and advanced periodontitis. Beube would later become the head of periodontics. He came to the United States from Canada, where he earned a DDS degree in 1930 at the University of Toronto. Dean Rappleye reported in his 1936 annual report that members of the oral diagnostic faculty were studying patients in the sterility clinic who had received injections of estrogenic and gonadotropic hormones and the effects of those hormones on gingivae and oral mucous membranes.

Charles Bodecker carried out fundamental studies on the structure of dental enamel. Bodecker had studied in Berlin with Rudolf Virchow and Nobel laureate Robert Koch. His classic studies of the nature of tooth structure led to advances in the knowledge and prevention of dental caries. Bodecker was joined by Edmund Applebaum and William Lefkowitz, both focusing on fluid movement in dentine. Bodecker also developed the Bodecker caries index, which was a progenitor of the Decayed, Missing, Filled (DMF) index, an index used today in national studies on dental caries.

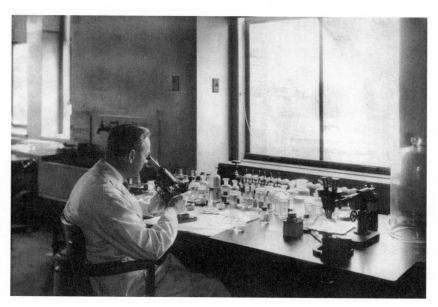

FIGURE 1.14 Dr. Edmund Applebaum, DDS, NYU 1922, (ca. 1930) was the second director of the oral histology research laboratory, established by Dr. Charles Bodecker in 1917. The laboratory has remained—albeit with updated equipment—up until the present, with Dr. Letty Moss-Salentijn as the director.

***

The merger of the Columbia University School of Dentistry with the freestanding College of Dental and Oral Surgery of New York to form the School of Dental and Oral Surgery on July 1, 1923, created a rich environment for the school's faculty to build its education and research programs. These studies continued on into the 1940s, but it appears that the war years made it difficult for the faculty to keep up teaching and research, especially since there was a shortage of full-time faculty due to the war and a shift to a faculty-intensive three-year curriculum in order to graduate students more quickly for the war effort.

CHAPTER TWO

1941–1978: Living Up to Standards

The Difficult Years

The second period in the history of the College of Dental Medicine is characterized by a protracted controversy over the merger of the School of Dental and Oral Surgery into the Faculty of Medicine. Circa 1944, President Nicholas Murray Butler explained the impending merger in the following way: "The new plan at Columbia University is designed to integrate the training for the two professions of dentistry and medicine as completely as possible without handicapping the development of either in its respective field of education, research and practice."[1] Although easily defined by Butler, the implementation of the merger created complex accreditation consequences, exacerbated by the faculty shortages that resulted from World War II.

The formal merger of the dental school into the medical faculty lasted from 1945 to 1959. As you may recall, Willard Rappleye, MD, served as the dean of both the medical and dental schools from 1933. When Dean Rappleye retired in 1958 the Faculty of Dentistry again separated from the Faculty of Medicine, and an independent school of dentistry, with its own dean, reemerged. As a result, accreditation difficulties were finally eased.

THE RAPPLEYE YEARS: AN OVERVIEW

Willard Rappleye was a Harvard Medical School graduate and a national leader in academic medicine. He became dean of the College of

Physicians and Surgeons at the age of thirty-eight after having held positions at the University of California, Yale, and Harvard. Rappleye was to become the longest-serving dean at P&S, serving for twenty-eight years from 1930 through 1958.

During his dual leadership, Rappleye created an administrative structure that included associate deans of dentistry, public health, and nursing under one faculty: the Faculty of Medicine. In the dental school, he delegated day-to-day operations to the associate dean.

After the tragic murder of Associate Dean Rowe in 1935, Houghton Holiday served as associate dean for ten years until Bion East took over in 1945. Maurice Hickey succeeded him in 1949. The relationships Rappleye had with these three associate deans—Holiday, East, and Hickey—were close ones. All had the same vision of dentistry as a close partner to medicine. The associate deans were in constant contact with Willard Rappleye, either through frequent meetings or via in-house written communications.

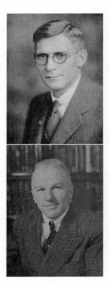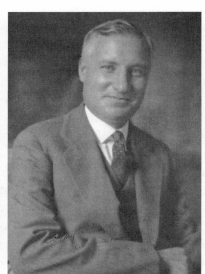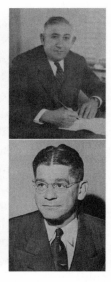

FIGURE 2.1 This composite photograph of Dean Willard Rappleye and the associate deans represents the administrative organization of the dental school to the medical school between 1935 and 1959. Rappleye (center) served as dean of both schools. Associate Deans Rowe (top left), Holiday (bottom left), East (top right), and Hickey (bottom right) ran day-to-day operations of the dental school.

Dean Rappleye's vision of dentistry as being closely aligned with medicine was clear and traced its roots to the founding document of the dental school. He indicated that oral surgery was already a specialty of medical practice and wrote, "The logical development would seem to be a closely articulated program for teaching in medicine and dentistry."[2] This was the position he steadfastly held throughout his deanship of both schools.

Under Rappleye's leadership, the dental school was administered through an administrative committee. In the 1941–1942 year, Dean Rappleye served as the committee's chair along with Associate Dean Holiday and six dental faculty professors: Charles Bodecker, Henry Sage Dunning, Leroy Hartman, Earle Hoyt, Harold Leonard, and Leuman Waugh. There was no problem with this type of administration up until the formal merger of the faculties in 1945, when the school became the School of Dental and Oral Surgery of the Faculty of Medicine. The formal merger led to a long dispute with the accrediting body, the American Dental Association's Council on Dental Education (CDE) now known as the Commission on Dental Accreditation.[3]

WITHDRAWAL OF APPROVED STATUS AND THE WORLD WAR II YEARS

Despite the clouds looming on the horizon, 1942 was a banner year for the dental school. The school celebrated its twenty-fifth year anniversary with a gala held at John Jay Hall. In the same year, the CDE found the school to be in excellent condition and it received full approval accreditation status.

However, this golden moment was to be short-lived. Just three years later, the merger controversy arose among the dental faculty. The faculty was divided over an internal resolution calling to restore an independent faculty of dentistry within Columbia University, rather than one administered under the dean of medicine, Willard Rappleye. Because the faculty was almost evenly divided on the resolution, Rappleye brought the matter to the administrative committee of the dental school. The committee decided that, as of February 5, 1945, the dental school should be fully integrated under the medical faculty. Shortly after, in October 1945, the CDE stated that it was suspending the school's approval status until it had an opportunity to reexamine the school. Two years later, on

August 1, 1947, the council terminated the school's approval status and dropped it from the list of approved dental schools mainly because of its merger and management by the medical school. Its reasoning was that the school lacked the same stature and independence of other schools within the University, as it did not have a separate faculty and control over its finances and appointment and promotion policies.

The University president stood behind the merger of the two schools and did not deviate from the original concept of the dental school as closely aligned to medicine. Dean Rappleye publicly stated that the CDE should not interfere with how dental schools were administered within the university, but should concentrate on the quality of the school. Just two years before the council's action to suspend the approval status, Rappleye pointed out that the school was rated as excellent by the council in all categories, including faculty, facilities, and the student body. What was especially upsetting to Columbia was that Harvard University around the same time announced that its dental school had become the School of Dental Medicine and would offer a five-year program leading to the combined degrees of DMD and MD. While Harvard never implemented the five-year combined degree program, the first two years of dental education were fully integrated with the medical school. Inexplicably, the CDE found no fault with that program.

As a consequence of the removal of the school's approval status by the CDE, between 1946 and 1948, the states of New Jersey, Pennsylvania, Connecticut, Vermont, and Maine refused to allow graduates from Columbia to be licensed in their states. Fortunately, however, New York did not follow suit—most of the students were New York State residents and the state needed the practitioners. So, for the moment, Columbia did not feel it needed to renege on what it believed to be its right to decide how to organize and integrate the school of dentistry into its structure.

Columbia was also justly proud of its graduates. In 1945, of thirty-six dental schools, its graduates had the third best performance on passing rates on the licensing exams. Forty-eight or 96 percent of Columbia's fifty graduates passed the licensing exam. Only graduates from the Universities of Nebraska and Minnesota did better.

THE SCHOOL MOVES FORWARD AND FUTURE
FACULTY GRADUATE

While the accreditation controversy festered, the leadership within the school, guided by the successive associate deans (Houghton Holiday, Bion East, and Maurice Hickey), kept the school moving forward. They advanced the predoctoral DDS, the postgraduate specialty certificate, and the dental hygiene programs.

Holiday served during the war years until 1944 when the school had a large number of students enrolled in the U.S. Army and Navy. The curriculum was accelerated by using summer sessions, allowing students to complete the four-year program in three calendar years. The war effort needed dentists and most dental schools shifted to three-year programs during World War II to assist the nation in educating the necessary workforce for the military. In 1944, thirty-eight of the dental school's graduates were commissioned as first lieutenants in the army and eight were commissioned as lieutenants (junior grade) in the Navy.

Dean Rappleye was proud of the cooperation and service that both the medical and dental schools provided to the military. According to Lou Mandel (DDS, SDOS 1946), there was much camaraderie among the medical and dental students who were in the Columbia military platoons. There were one dental student platoon and two medical student platoons. Each morning at 7:00 a.m., all of the students assembled in their uniforms in formation on Fort Washington Avenue in front of the Armory and marched around the Armory; once a month there was a formal review of the platoons in the Armory with a medal awarded for the best platoon. Competition for the medal between the platoons was strong. The students' tuitions and stipends of $54 per month were paid by the military during their school years.

Not surprisingly, enrollment fluctuated during the war years. There were fifty-one DDS graduates in 1941, of whom three already held the MD degrees and one received the MD and DDS through a special six-year program. By 1947 the number of DDS graduates had returned to the prewar average of forty. However, entering enrollment increased once again in 1949 to fifty-two students due to the great need for dentists. The dentist-to-population ratio was approximately 1:2,200, far

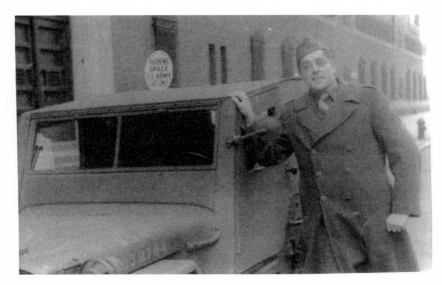

FIGURE 2.2 Dr. Louis Mandel (ca. 1943) was a student at SDOS during the World War II years. Here he is shown in uniform as he served in the dental school army platoon. The Armory on 168th Street is shown in the background.

above the number of patients that dentists could treat, given the high level of dental disease during that prefluoride time.

The school's income from fees and tuition grew to $227,425 ($2.7 million in 2014 dollars) by 1946. Income from "infirmary fees" (today we call this clinic income) was $105,000 ($1.3 million in 2014 dollars), while tuition from the DDS, Postdoctoral, and dental hygiene programs combined was $119,325 ($1.5 million in 2014 dollars). Fees for clinical procedures in 1949 ranged from $2 to $6 for an amalgam restoration to $11 for a full gold crown ($20, $59, and $107, respectively, in current dollars). An orthodontic case cost about $288 per year or $24 per month ($2,865 and $238, respectively, in current dollars).

During the 1940s, SDOS graduates joined the faculty. The timing was such that these graduates became the bridge from the faculty formed in the early years of the school—who were reaching retirement age—to the future. Most of this second wave of faculty served well into the 1980s. Joseph Leavitt, class of 1940, helped establish the specialty field of endodontics and became the first director of the endodontic division at Columbia in the mid-1960s. Irving Naidorf, a 1941 graduate, would become an assistant dean for postgraduate programs and a national leader in the field of endodontics. Nicholas DiSalvo, a member of the class of 1942, went on to earn a PhD and would become the director of the Division of Orthodontics. Henry Nahoum, class of 1943, joined the faculty as an assistant and then full time in the 1950s in the division of orthodontics. Robert Gottsegen, class of 1943 and graduate of the first class in the periodontics postdoctoral program in 1948, became the director of the Division of Periodontics, a position he held until retirement.

Irwin Mandel was a 1945 graduate and served on the faculty first as a research assistant and then later in the late 1960s as a full-time faculty member. Herbert Bartelstone, also in the class of 1945, earned a PhD degree in pharmacology and eventually became associate dean of the dental school in the early 1970s. Edward Cain, class of 1945, would become the director of operative dentistry and served as associate dean for academic affairs in the late 1970s.

Five members of the class of 1946 joined the faculty: Louis Mandel, George Minervini, John Piro, Solon (Art) Ellison, and Melvin Moss. Ellison and Moss stayed on to earn PhD degrees in the fellowship program in the basic sciences. Lou Mandel earned a certificate in oral surgery and, with George Minervini, became codirector of the Division of Oral Surgery. John Piro became director of the maxillofacial prosthetics program at Memorial Sloan Kettering Hospital and served for a while as interim director of the Division of Prosthodontics at Columbia. Ellison went on to become a leader at the State University of New York in Buffalo. Moss became dean of the dental school at Columbia. Lou Mandel remained at Columbia in the oral surgery division and as of 2015 remains an active member of the faculty and associate dean for hospital programs (see also Chapter 5). John Lucca, who graduated in 1947, would become the director of prosthodontics.

Looking back, it was quite remarkable that so many of the future leaders of the dental school would be drawn from these classes. These individuals, supported by a stellar group of loyal and talented part-time faculty drawn from the greater New York City area, kept the school moving forward during difficult times. As mentioned earlier, while this group was joining the faculty, many long-time faculty from the founding days were retiring or leaving the school. For example, William Dunning

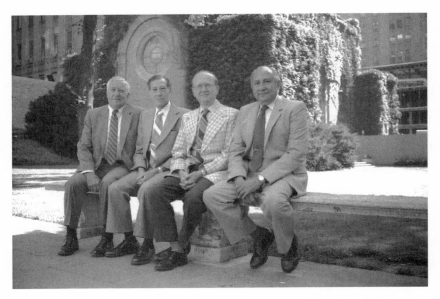

FIGURE 2.3 A photograph from the 1980s of four faculty members from classes that graduated in the 1940s. Sitting on a bench in the Medical Center Garden from left to right are: George Minervini (class of 1946), Henry Nahoum (class of 1943), Nicholas DiSalvo (class of 1942), and John Lucca (class of 1947).

retired from practice in 1946. A dinner in his honor was held at the Men's Faculty Club on West 117th Street. Around this same time, Henry Gillett passed away and Isador Hirschfeld retired.

THE POSTGRADUATE AND THE DENTAL HYGIENE PROGRAMS ADVANCE

On March 6, 1945, Bion East was appointed associate dean of the dental school—news that was big enough to be reported in the *New York Times*. Thus, East was in the challenging position of following through on the new plan to integrate the dental school into the medical faculty. Bion East received his DDS training at the University of Michigan, receiving his degree in 1908. East had served in France during World War I and was director of the dental service at a base hospital. Prior to his appointment as an assistant professor at the Columbia-affiliated De Lamar Institute of Public Health, he was the consulting oral surgeon at the U. S. Public Health Service from 1922 to 1933.

East represented the type of leader Gies had envisioned for Columbia. In his landmark report, Gies had indicated that the scope, complexity, and medical demands on dentistry made it impossible for any one practitioner to be an expert in all aspects of dentistry and that postgraduate studies were needed. Columbia became a leader in creating postgraduate opportunities, beginning in 1927 with the postgraduate program in orthodontics and then later with postgraduate course work in the basic sciences, clinical dentistry, and dental hygiene. Rappleye noted in his annual report that by 1940 a greater number of graduates each year elected to enter into internships in hospitals and that the dental school encouraged that movement. Clearly, there was a demand for courses beyond the short continuing education courses the school offered. East recognized that dentistry and dental hygiene needed advanced education opportunities for graduates. During his tenure he advanced the postgraduate programs, furthering their growth.

When it came to another matter, East was not so successful. He understood the need to enhance the research agenda and looked toward the National Institutes of Health for funding. In turn, NIH requested an endorsement from Columbia for a bill to establish the National Institute of Dental Research. However, when East turned to Rappleye for the endorsement, Rappleye said he was not in favor of such an institute and instead the funds should go directly to the schools of dentistry.

SDOS BECOMES AN EARLY LEADER IN POSTGRADUATE EDUCATION FOR DENTISTS

SDOS had a rich history in postgraduate specialty education programs, which began with the absorption of the New York Post-graduate School in 1917. In 1941 there were already thirty-seven dentists enrolled in postdoctoral programs, of whom twenty-five were in the orthodontic certificate program and one in the oral surgery certificate program. For example, Isador Hirschfeld stated the case for periodontics to be a specialty in an article in the yearbook of 1940. By 1947 certificates were being granted in advanced courses in oral surgery, general dentistry, and periodontology, all of which joined the long-standing advanced education program in orthodontics. The periodontic postdoctoral program was among one of the first such programs organized in the country.

SDOS was also a leader in the field of pedodontics (now called pediatric dentistry). In 1929 Ewing Cleveland McBeath (DDS, University of Minnesota 1910, and MD, University of Minnesota 1921) was recruited to Columbia by Alfred Owre to establish a division of pedodontics. By 1950 he had established a postgraduate certificate program in pedodontics, one of the earliest such programs in the world. By 1950 there were twenty-nine postgraduate certificates issued, nineteen in orthodontics, four in oral surgery, four in periodontics, and two in general dentistry. Postgraduate certificate programs in prosthodontics were added, and then an endodontic postgraduate certificate program established in 1966 became another early program under the leadership of Joseph Leavitt and Irving Naidorf. However, in the 1970s, the postgraduate certificate programs in prosthodontics and oral surgery were no longer offered. The loss of operating room privileges made it impossible to continue the oral surgery residency program. Both programs would return as postdoctoral programs at SDOS in the 1980s.

The school began landmark fellowship programs for DDS graduates in the following basic science departments: anatomy, bacteriology, biochemistry, pathology, pharmacology, and physiology. The University accepted thirty points toward the PhD degree for the work done under the professional degree. Five graduates from the classes in the 1940s who wished to become faculty scholars were accepted into this program.[4] This was the first such fellowship program for dentists in the United States. Including dentists who had earned the PhD in the various basic science fields in these departments ensured that research in dentistry would remain at the same high level as that in medicine. All of the individuals identified above who completed the PhD programs played prominent roles in the dental school at Columbia, except Solon (Art) Ellison, who was recruited to be the founding chair of a new department of oral biology at the State University of New York at Buffalo. Between 1963 and 1976, under his leadership, this first department of oral biology in the United States reached great prominence in research and in educating future researchers. Ellison returned to Columbia in 1976 to serve on the dental school faculty.

In addition to the certificate specialty programs and the doctoral programs in the basic sciences, there was a one-year course leading to a master of science degree in public health. The school even offered fellowships of $2,000 ($24,100 in 2014 dollars) for graduates interested in pursuing research in prevention.

THE DENTAL HYGIENE PROGRAM
CONTINUES TO GROW

In 1947 the Dental Hygiene Program supported by Bion East began requiring two years of college prior to enrollment in the two-year dental hygiene program. The university approved the school's proposal, strongly supported by Bion East and later by Houghton Holiday, to award the bachelor of science degree to the graduates.

As the 1930s closed and the 1940s began, the dental hygiene program was graduating about forty students per year. They were gaining clinical experience at three locations: The students treated 1,975 patients in the Medical Center adult clinic; 1,705 patients (mostly Columbia faculty and personnel) in the Pupin Physics Laboratory on the Morningside campus; and 2,125 children at the children's clinic at 15 Amsterdam Avenue. In 1948 Dr. Louise Ball, the faculty member who founded the dental hygiene program at Columbia, passed away, and Frances A. Stoll, RDH, MA, became the director of the program. Dr. Ball left the dental school a bequest of $50,000 ($403,000 in 2014 dollars). She also left $500,000, or almost $5 million in current dollars, to the dental school at Howard University, where she had been a member of the board of trustees, as well as a close friend of the dean of the dental school, and had helped set up the dental hygiene program with a Columbia graduate as head of the program.

By the end of the decade, Dean Rappleye raised the funds needed to build additional floors to the Vanderbilt Clinic above what is now the ninth floor and which was then the top floor of the building. There was discussion about the dental school expanding and taking another floor above its space, but that never happened. When Bion East left in 1948 to take up the reins of the Veterans Administration Dental Service, Maurice Hickey became the associate dean for dentistry, still under the merged faculty. Hickey, a DMD graduate of the Harvard Dental School in 1932, had earned his MD degree at Columbia in 1927. He served through the 1950s, while the school was still part of the Faculty of Medicine.

THE 1950S: THE HICKEY YEARS

In 1950, some five years after the suspension and subsequent with-drawal of the approval classification of the dental school, Columbia was informing applicants that some states would not grant licenses to Columbia degree holders. The University's president and the dean of the medical and dental school, Willard Rappleye, were still adamant that the CDE should not dictate how the University structured the administra-tion of its programs. In fact, the states' sentiments seemed to be turning. New Jersey, which had previously announced that it would not license Columbia graduates because the dental school lacked CDE accredi-tation, did a turnabout. It restored the Columbia SDOS to the list of approved dental schools, stating that minor administrative differences should not affect a school when trained dentists are in demand. New York State continued to back the Columbia program completely.

After becoming associate dean in 1950, Maurice Hickey recognized that times were changing for dentistry and for the school. For example, the NIH had set up the National Institute of Dental Research, water fluoridation was becoming widespread, the demand for dental care became greater from advances in prevention and treatment, and new public dental schools were being created by states in which dentists were needed.

Hickey moved quickly to resolve the lingering accreditation prob-lem. He invited the CDE to return to the school for another visit in Janu-ary of 1951. After that evaluation, the council wrote to the then president of Columbia, Dwight D. Eisenhower, that as of February 2, 1951, the dental school was back on the approved list. In the council's letter to Eisenhower, the secretary of the Council of Dental Education reported that the members of the visiting committee said that "the position of the School of Dental and Oral Surgery in the administrative structure of Columbia University is quite unlike that of other dental schools in this country . . . emphasized by the fact that the [school] is academically the Department of Dentistry of the Faculty of Medicine. . . . The dental school should have stature, recognition, and acceptance by the univer-sity on the same terms as other professional schools in the university." The report went on to indicate that the undergraduate dental education program "is being conducted in such a manner that it is accomplishing its goal of training and educating qualified dental graduates and, on this basis, [the council] recommends approval." However, the letter went on to state that the visiting committee "is also of the opinion that appropriate modifications of the administrative nomenclature and structure would be extremely helpful in clarifying the position dental instruction has in Columbia University."

The council had changed its view on the Columbia administrative structure. This was big news. In fact, *The New York Times* covered the story on February 17, 1951, with the headline: "Dentistry Rating Won by Columbia—Rappleye Hails Ties with Medicine, Public Health and Nursing." Rappleye's point that dentistry, nursing, and public health were logically all part of the medical profession and should be under "one roof" was finally vindicated. But even though the accreditation status was restored, the dental faculty and the dental alumni were still unhappy with the arrangement. They wanted more autonomy. Some claimed there was a conflict of interest within the administrative structure because the dean of the medical school had too much power, especially in making decisions about resources that could advantageously affect the medical school.

The Hickey years (1945–1956) were, nevertheless, good years for the dental school. The 1950s saw a big demand for dentists. The *New York Times* reported on the Columbia conference to feature the painless drill called the Cavitron, which Carol Oman, director of operative dentistry, and Edmund Applebaum, a noted faculty researcher, had tested and found to be suitable for cavity preparation. The Council for Cerebral Palsy funded two graduate fellowships to study how to manage the treatment of cerebral palsy patients. Later, a special two-chair clinic was also funded for such care under the direction of the pedodontic division. By 1956 more than 46,000 patient visits were recorded in the dental clinic.

The school's dental museum, originally headed by Henry Gillett, was rededicated as the Charles H. Land Museum. Land was the grandfather of Colonel Charles Lindbergh and a dentist who pioneered in the use of porcelain in dentistry. Dr. Curt Proskauer was the curator of the museum at the time and served in that role from 1951 to 1965. The Land collection and the rest of the school's museum collection were later donated by Columbia to the Smithsonian, and the school's museum was closed.

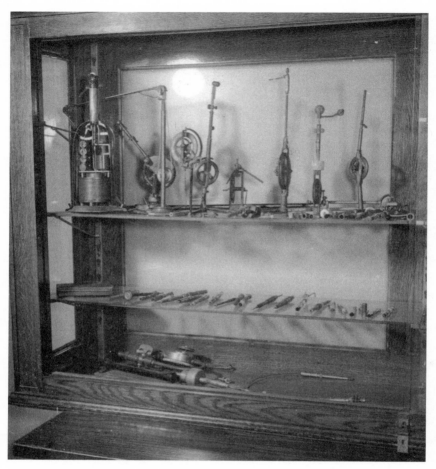

FIGURE 2.4 The School of Dental and Oral Surgery housed a dental museum. Several cases such as this one held early instruments and dental drills. Dr. Curt Proskauer was the curator of the museum until Columbia's collection was donated to the Smithsonian Museum.

Frances Stoll, the director of the dental hygiene program, wrote to Associate Dean Hickey that there was now a growing need for dental hygienists to earn master's degrees because so many of the Columbia graduates were being recruited to head up dental hygiene programs throughout the United States. In fact 50 percent of the graduating class of 1952 was recruited to teaching and administration positions. Stoll did not believe they were adequately trained for that role and was able

ALUMNI VOICES: JOAN PHELAN

Joan Phelan, DDS, received her BS in 1962 and MS in 1967 from the dental hygiene programs at Columbia. She recalls that her interest in dentistry began from a discussion while in college with her lab partner in zoology who was going to enter the dental hygiene program. Dr. Phelan, who an English major in college, says, "I had never heard of dental hygiene as a career." However, "the more I learned about dental hygiene, the more interested I became. So at the beginning of my junior college year in 1960, I entered the baccalaureate dental hygiene program at Columbia University."

She vividly remembers her class upon entering the two-year dental hygiene training program as "a class of thirteen single girls" who lived in Johnson Hall on the Morningside campus, and who took the subway to 168th Street. The director of the program, Dr. Francis Stoll, "did everything possible to separate the dental hygiene students from the dental students . . . all our

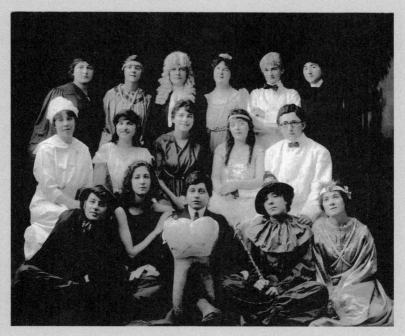

FIGURE 2.5 Dental hygiene students were not encouraged to fraternize with the dental students. This all-female class had to play the roles of men in their skit called "A War on Caries" (ca. 1917).

classes were separate from the dental students. We were not supposed to socialize with dental students on the medial center campus . . . [in truth] there was a lot of socializing outside the Medical Center campus—but none of my classmates married a dental student."

After graduating from the dental hygiene program, getting married, and moving to Michigan, Phelan worked as a dental hygienist and then later as an elementary school teacher. After returning to New York City in 1965, she was invited to return to Columbia for the new master's degree program in dental hygiene, which was then under the direction of Ms. Patricia McLean.

Things had changed under McLean. There was much more interaction with dental students and even joint classes with them. One of them was the oral pathology course taught by Edward Zegarelli. Other courses were at Teachers College. Upon completion of the master's degree program, Phelan practiced dental hygiene and taught at the dental hygiene program at State University of New York, Farmingdale.

The road to dental school was next for her. However, she recalls that when she was attending her first dental hygiene program at Columbia, Dr. Francis Stoll dissuaded the hygiene students from continuing future career directions by "making it a point to tell us that women do not make good dentists!" How the world has changed!

Joan Phelan was accepted into the inaugural DMD class at the SUNY Stony Brook School of Dental Medicine. She then completed a residency in oral pathology; perhaps her interest in that field was stimulated in the class Edward Zegarelli taught to both hygiene and dental students. Dr. Phelan has had a successful career in dentistry and is a well-respected educator and oral and maxillofacial pathologist. Today she is professor and chair of the Department of Oral and Maxillofacial Pathology, Radiology and Medicine at the New York University College of Dentistry.

to develop, along with Hickey, the master of science in dental hygiene degree program by April of 1953. It was soon approved, and Columbia graduates continued to be sought to start new dental hygiene programs across the country.

Big changes were about to happen as the Hickey era and the 1950s came to a close. In 1956, Maurice Hickey was recruited to become the dean at the University of Washington School of Dentistry in Seattle. Two years later in 1958, Willard Rappleye retired, after twenty-eight years as dean of the medical school and fifteen years as dean of the medical and dental schools.

H. Houston Merritt succeeded Rappleye, and Gilbert Smith succeeded Hickey in 1956 as associate dean. Merritt had been chair of neurology and was well known for his work on anticonvulsant therapy and the use of Dilantin to control epilepsy. Gilbert Smith, a longtime faculty member who received his dental degree from the University of Minnesota in 1927, was the director of prosthetic dentistry at the time of his appointment as associate dean. Smith presided over the return of the dental school to an independent faculty and the restoration of the administration of the school, with the top administrative officer being the dean.

These major administrative changes were recommended in 1957 by the President's Committee on the Educational Future of the University, which stated that the dental school should have its own dean and faculty; a status that would allow it to stand beside the medical school under the general direction of the vice president in charge of medical affairs. Two years later, in 1959, the University's trustees approved the proposal, creating two faculties on the medical campus, the Faculty of Medicine and the Faculty of Dental and Oral Surgery. A University press release on February 23, 1957, quoted President Grayson Kirk saying he recognized "the increasingly important role of dentistry in the health sciences," and that the action "was taken with the object of stimulating the growth of dental education and research in the University." In addition, Kirk stated that "the present close relationship of the medical and dental faculties with respect to instruction of dental students will continue."[5]

Gilbert Smith now was dean of the SDOS, returning to the administrative structure that existed when Alfred Owre was dean in the 1930s. A new chapter was opening up in the 1960s, one that would bring new accreditation problems, similar to those that had characterized the Rappleye years and the Hickey era.

THE 1960S: A NEW ERA IN THE DENTAL SCHOOL

Now, with its new independence from the Faculty of Medicine and under its fully restored dean and a cadre of faculty leaders appointed from the ranks of the 1940s graduates, the school could more easily map

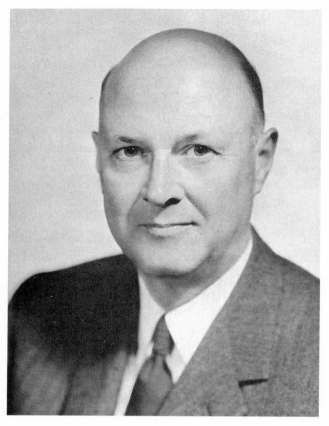

FIGURE 2.6 Dr. Gilbert Smith (DDS, University of Minnesota 1927) served as the associate dean under the Rappleye administration from 1956 until he became dean in 1959, when Houston Merritt succeeded Rappleye and the dental school became independent of the medical school.

out its own destiny. But it was not going to be easy. The class size in 1960 was still about forty DDS students. There were sixty-three postgraduate students in four specialty programs: periodontics, pedodontics, oral surgery, and orthodontics (the largest).

The dental hygiene program was enrolling thirty-three students into its baccalaureate and master's programs. In the midst of this growth, Frances Stoll retired as director of the dental hygiene program and was replaced in 1965 by Patricia McLean, who continued this forward movement. McLean had earned her certificate in dental hygiene at Columbia, a baccalaureate degree from New York University, and a master's degree in administration at Columbia. She was born in Buffalo, New York, and was the daughter of a dentist.

The DDS program continued to evolve. A new senior rotation at Roosevelt Hospital was instituted in which students were on call, served in the emergency clinic and the hospital dental clinic, gained experience in the operating room, and learned venipuncture. The dental school also affiliated with six other hospitals: Mount Sinai, Montefiore, Bronx Veterans, Grasslands, Long Island, and Long Island Jewish. Through the strong leadership of Joseph Leavitt, a new two-year certificate post-graduate program in endodontics was established. The oral surgery

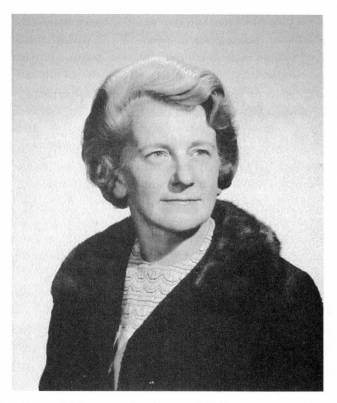

FIGURE 2.7 Patricia McLean served as director of the Division of Dental Hygiene from 1965 to 1977. Dean Edward Zegarelli appointed her as an assistant dean prior to her retirement.

postdoctoral program increased from two to three years in length. The school entered into an agreement to provide 1,000 hours of a didactic program in applied basic sciences spread over the three years of training for six oral surgery programs at hospitals in the New York City area. The hospitals included Presbyterian and Delafield (New York City's cancer hospital adjacent to the Medical Center campus) and four of the six hospitals with which the school was affiliated. In 1966 the school's clinics treated 17,942 patients and the orthodontic clinic had 477 cases under treatment.

But troubles with the CDE reemerged. As the result of a 1963 visit by the accrediting team, the dental school was placed on provisional accreditation. This time, the council cited insufficient facilities, a lack of full-time faculty, and inadequate representation of the dental faculty on important Medical Center committees as critical issues. The school was given two years to rectify the problems.

These problems had been long-standing and were recognized by the vice president in charge of medical affairs and the president of the University. In fact, as early as May 1945, Willard Rappleye had sent a letter to Nicholas Murray Butler about the facilities problem, noting that the dental school was operating under great handicaps because of the lack of space. It was apparent again in 1957 that the dental school needed to have larger facilities. There was insufficient research space and not enough support space for academic and clinical programs. Since the 1950s, discussions had been underway in the University to plan for a new building for the dental school. An ad hoc committee of the University trustees was set up to review the problems in the dental school and recognized that the dental school's issues could be resolved. After serious study they also held that they "ardently champion the continuation of the Dental School and strongly favor its association with the Medical Center."[6]

The dental school had some preliminary plans drawn up for a new building at an estimated cost of $6 million ($51 million in 2014 dollars). However, Dean Rappleye and President Grayson Kirk thought it would actually cost $10 million ($85 million in 2014 dollars) to build a new dental school. The dental school started its first fund-raising campaign around this time, but $10 million seemed to be a difficult reach for the school. However, there were funds available from the government for construction and there were statements of support from the University for the school to proceed in planning a new building. The University was investigating the possibility of using air rights over the Armory or of building on land it owned in the Medical Center location.

In the midst of these issues, Gilbert Smith, who had maintained a busy private practice while being dean, decided that he wanted to step down to pursue practice full time. This meant that attention was diverted from planning for a new dental school building in the mid-1960s toward finding a replacement for Gilbert Smith. Smith had brought the school its hard-won independence from the medical school. The new dean would be faced with accreditation problems as well as rejuvenating an aging facility, representing the school in the Medical Center, and hiring more full-time faculty. The ad hoc trustee committee and the accrediting committee also criticized the lack of research activity at the school— an important issue, since the Gies legacy had long held to the principle of research being an integral part of the faculty's responsibilities.

1968–1978: A TIME OF TRANSITION

Even though the dental school was experiencing some major internal problems surrounding space, accreditation, and personnel changes, the decade of the 1960s became known as the golden age for health science research and for the expansion of medical and dental schools in the United States. The federal government developed legislation that encouraged schools to expand enrollment and made funds available for facilities for existing and new schools. Dental schools became eligible to apply for funds from the National Institute of Dental Research to form dental research centers. The five schools funded were able to build strong research programs. Unfortunately, SDOS was not among those five schools.

Gilbert Smith's resignation in 1968 prompted Houston Merritt, the vice president in charge of medical affairs and dean of P&S, to visit with the director of the National Institute of Dental Research. He reported to President Grayson Kirk that his visit indicated that Columbia's selection of a full-time dean was critical to the future of the school. The application for federal funds to rebuild the facility and for research would be largely dependent on the appointment of such a person. Additionally, the school needed an individual who could work with the accrediting council to move the school from provisional to full accreditation, recruit full-time faculty, and improve relationships of the school with the hospital and medical faculty.

1968–1978: MELVIN MOSS AND EDWARD ZEGARELLI LEAD THE SCHOOL

Between 1968 and 1978, the University turned to two of its own to tackle the issues. Melvin Moss (DDS, SDOS 1946, and PhD, Graduate School of Arts and Sciences 1954) was appointed dean in 1968 and served until 1973. He was followed by Edward Zegarelli (DDS, SDOS 1937), who remained in that position until 1978. Each man, in his own way, set out to tackle the issues of finances, facilities, and faculty growth during the greatest period of social change in the United States.

During this period, P&S and the administrative structure of the Medical Center also underwent change. Paul Marks (MD, P&S 1949), became dean of the medical school and vice president for medical affairs in 1970. In 1973 the combined position of vice president and dean of the medical school were temporarily separated. Marks continued in the renamed position of vice president for health sciences, and Donald Tapley was appointed dean of P&S. Their leadership supported the progress needed in the dental school.

Born in Manhattan, Melvin Moss was a New Yorker through and through. He received his AB at New York University in 1942 before going on to earn his DDS at SDOS and his PhD in anatomy. He held a postdoctoral fellowship from the U.S. Public Health Service, served in the Army Dental Corps, and then joined the P&S faculty in the Department of Anatomy. Moss was a dynamic lecturer and generations of medical and dental students found him to be an outstanding teacher. His research and publications on the functional matrix explained growth and development of the human skull. The functional matrix has become a mainstay in the field of orthodontics and assists treatment regimes. Upon being appointed as dean in 1968, Moss laid out a plan to the University to improve staffing, update the curriculum, and renovate the main clinical facility. He also investigated the potential for a new building for the school.

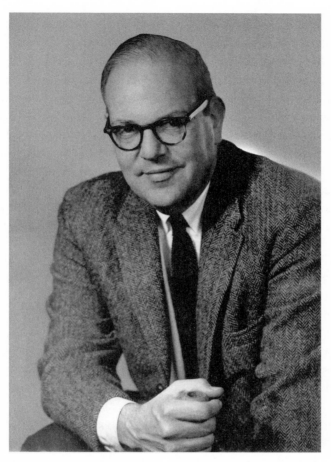

FIGURE 2.8 Dr. Melvin Moss served as the dean of SDOS from 1968 to 1973.
He graduated with a DDS from SDOS in 1946 and earned a PhD from the Columbia
Graduate School of Arts and Sciences in 1954. He returned to the Department of
Anatomy upon completing his term as dean.

Moss appointed Herbert Bartelstone, another Columbia alumnus, as
associate dean. Bartelstone graduated from SDOS in 1946 and earned his
PhD in Pharmacology at P&S in 1960. A member of the pharmacology
department, he also conducted a busy private practice and treated complex cases requiring major prosthodontic rehabilitation of the dentition.
Working together, Moss and Bartelstone sought to resolve the accreditation issues by bringing the school's clinical curriculum up to date and

expanding the research program. In addition to the core basic science program taught jointly to medical and dental students, earlier introduction to clinical dentistry in the first two years included subjects in preventive dentistry, psychological aspects of patient care, and correlation clinics to integrate the clinical aspects of care with the basic sciences and clinic observation in the second year. Modes of instruction now included small-group teaching and upper-class students serving as preceptors to those in the classes below them. Electives were introduced into the fourth year, and summer clinic sessions were added for all students. This was quite a departure from the usual dental school curriculum, in which students received little to no introduction to patient care until the third year of dental school. In addition, the school would strengthen its research program through the addition of new full-time faculty.

Moss appointed three full-time professors: Irwin Mandel as director of the new Division of Preventive Dentistry, Sidney Horowitz to head up the Division of Growth and Development, and Robert Gottsegen (brought back from the University of Pennsylvania) as director of periodontics. These three new full-time professors enhanced the faculty, which at the time had only eighteen full-time members, and began the process of expanding research and bringing new ideas into the faculty at a critical time in dental education.

These initial steps and newly appointed full-time faculty led the school to advance further into the national mainstream of dental education during the changing times of the 1960s. One of these advances was a system of course evaluation, started by Samuel Dworkin, who was appointed to the faculty in 1970. In 1972 he set up the Office of Education and Behavioral Science—an innovation at the time. Dworkin (DDS, NYU 1958, and PhD in clinical psychology, NYU 1969) studied the psychosocial factors in oral disease and pain responses with James Lipton (DDS, SDOS 1971, and Columbia PhD, 1980), who was a graduate student at the time. Both Dworkin and Lipton would become distinguished in their fields, Dworkin at the University of Washington and Lipton at the National Institute of Dental and Craniofacial Research and at the University of Pennsylvania. (A profile of James Lipton can be found in Chapter 6.)

Irwin Mandel, an SDOS graduate in 1945, joined the faculty in 1946 as a research assistant and part-time faculty member before joining the

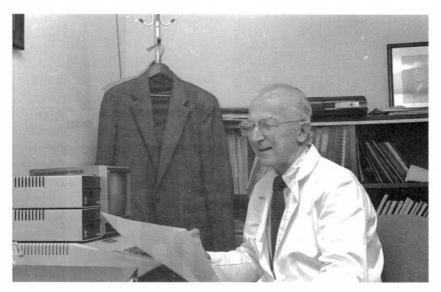

FIGURE 2.9 Dr. Sidney Horowitz was recruited to Columbia by Melvin Moss to head up a Division of Growth and Development. A 1945 DDS graduate of NYU, he earned a certificate in orthodontics at SDOS in 1949. He later became associate dean for academic affairs under the administration of Dean Allan Formicola.

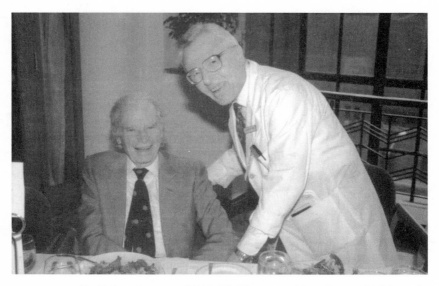

FIGURE 2.10 Dr. Robert Gottsegen (DDS, SDOS 1943, and Periodontics, SDOS 1948) returned to Columbia to head up the Division of Periodontics. Here he is shown (right) with his predecessor, Dr. Frank Beube. Both men were pioneers in the field of periodontics.

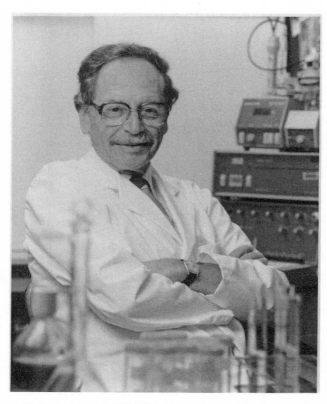

FIGURE 2.11 Dr. Irwin Mandel (DDS, SDOS 1945) joined the faculty as a research assistant in 1946. He became a full-time faculty member recruited by Dean Moss in the 1970s. Mandel was the first recipient of the American Dental Association's Gold Medal for Excellence in Dental Research in 1985.

faculty full time in 1968. He founded the Division of Preventive Dentistry in 1971, the first such division in the country, and infused the curriculum with course work in prevention of oral disease. He was a well-known clinician-scientist who was the first recipient of the American Dental Association's gold medal award for Excellence in Dental Research. His research on dental caries attracted continuous funding from the National Institute of Dental Research.

Sidney Horowitz (DDS, New York University 1945, and SDOS Orthodontics 1949) was recruited from NYU where he had been the associate director of the cleft palate program. At Columbia he established the Division of Orofacial Growth and Development and pioneered important research in craniofacial anomalies and their treatment. Robert Gottsegen (DDS, SDOS 1943 and SDOS Periodontics 1948) researched the relationship between diabetes and periodontal disease. He rose to become the president of the American Academy of Periodontics, 1970–1971.

The relationship between the medical and dental schools and how faculty mentors influenced career directions are highlighted in the story of Dr. Michael Barnett, now retired, who looks back on his student years at SDOS during the 1960s.

ALUMNI VOICES: MICHAEL BARNETT

Michael Barnett received his DDS degree from SDOS in 1967. He completed his predental requirements in three years at Columbia College. Barnett says, "One could say that Columbia is in my genes." Two of his cousins also graduated from Columbia College, and one of them, Robert Loring (formerly Lifschutz), graduated from SDOS in 1958 and the orthodontic program in 1963. In the 1920s Barnett's uncle, Alex Lifschutz, also graduated from the dental school and later served as president of the alumni association in 1957–1958. While it was almost inevitable that Barnett would not break family tradition and would come to SDOS, he cites "a relatively small class size [forty] and the school's close association with the medical school resulting in a rigorous basic science education" as other reasons for selecting Columbia. This hallmark of the Columbia Dental School from its inception continues today and is cited by students in the present time as a reason for selecting the school.

Regarding his educational experience at the school in the mid-1960s, Barnett credits the "close relationship and interaction with the medical school" and "certain faculty who provided examples and inspiration for individuals, such as myself who were drawn to the more biologically based aspects of clinical practice . . ." as influencing his career direction.

He looked up to faculty members Irwin Mandel and Herbert Bartelstone. He calls Mandel a "research superstar" focusing on studies of the role of saliva in maintaining oral health and function. Bartlestone, an SDOS graduate who also held the PhD degree and was a member of the pharmacology department in P&S, combined a successful research career while also conducting a "high-end restorative practice on the East Side" according to Barnett. Bartlestone invited Barnett to spend a day in his office, and that solidified the notion for him that one could pursue research while still practicing dentistry.

While a dental student, Barnett had the opportunity to hold summer fellowships in the cardiac physiology laboratory of P&S. Dr. Austin (Bill) Kutscher, a faculty member in what was then known as the stomatology department (today called oral diagnosis), helped develop his interest in oral medicine and clinical oral pathology. All of this led Barnett into what he calls a "very untraditional career path," especially "for the time at which I graduated."

With an NIH training grant, Barnett continued his studies in oral pathology at the University of Washington but was interrupted in those studies by serving in the U.S. Army as Chief of Oral Medicine during the Vietnam War years. While he was in the military, his interest grew in the field of periodontics, and he later pursued a three-year postdoctoral program at Harvard University designed for graduate dentists who wished to follow an academic career path. Subsequently, Barnett served on the faculty of periodontics at the University of Medicine and Dentistry of New Jersey, SUNY Buffalo, and the University of Louisville.

He notes that he was hired in New Jersey by Allan Formicola, who was department chair there and "who continued to serve as a mentor and friend throughout my subsequent career."

After leaving Louisville, Barnett was recruited to chair the department of dentistry at the Morristown Memorial Hospital in New Jersey while also serving as general practice residency program director. He was later recruited by the Warner-Lambert Company to serve as associate director of dental affairs and then as senior director, overseeing a large research team. For a number of years many of the readers of this book will remember Mike Barnett's articles in the *Journal of the American Dental Association* in which he summarized recent research findings.

Barnett sums up his unusual career path this way, "When I graduated in 1967 I could never have envisioned the path my career would take and the varied types of positions I would have over the years. While my DDS from Columbia provided a starting point, subsequent events enabled me to branch out and have a career that provided variety and the ability . . . no, the necessity . . . of constantly learning new things along the way." The founders of the Columbia University Dental School had in mind that the school would provide such a foundation for its graduates and enrich the field of dentistry for the benefit of the public, as has Mike Barnett.

Finally, during this time period, a far-reaching plan of community dentistry was developed by Harold Applewhite (DDS, MPH). The plan envisioned a mobile van to reach schoolchildren in Washington Heights and off-site student rotations to community-serving facilities. Decades earlier, in the 1920s, Frank Thorn Van Woert and Louise Ball had also proposed plans to reach schoolchildren. However, it would have to wait until the 1990s for the school to actually implement a plan to provide preventive care and treatment to schoolchildren in need.

Moss was able to gain funding to improve the existing facility in Vanderbilt Clinic through a $400,000 renovation and new equipment fund for the main dental clinic. He also explored options for expanding the existing space and eventually building a new facility for the school. Some of the plans included obtaining the four basement floors of the then under construction Columbia Towers on Haven Avenue for office and research space; building a new dental school facility on top of the new building planned for the Augustus Long Health Sciences Library; and building a new building on sites east of Broadway. Eventually, an additional 7,500 square feet of space was made available for the use of the school in a building at 21 Audubon Avenue.

In 1970 Moss began what would become a long process of obtaining New York State aid for the private dental schools, that is, New York University and Columbia. New York State had already provided capitation aid for the private medical schools. The basis for the aid was to improve the shortage of physicians and dentists in the state. Moss appointed Stephen Wotman, DDS, as a special assistant. Wotman, with the assistance of Dr. Fred Putney, assistant vice president for medical affairs, did much of the analysis and background work for the development of New York State aid for the dental school. By 1972 the proposal had been further developed, and a bill to provide $1,500 per student in capitation support and $300,000 for facility improvement was placed on the table, but it still remained to be passed by the legislature.

Fortunately, after a site visit by the CDE in 1972, the progress on the issues that had placed the school on provisional accreditation status was sufficient for the school to receive full accreditation approval status. However, the school was still required to report progress on the CDE's recommendations. After serving for five years, Melvin Moss decided to step aside as dean in the summer of 1973. Moss felt that he had accomplished what needed to be done to solve the immediate accreditation problem and that he wished to return to his research and teaching career in the Department of Anatomy.[7] The coeditor of the alumni newsletter characterized Melvin Moss as "a type that only America could have produced. He is an amazing combination of dynamic executive and classic scholar in the finest tradition of Oxford, the Sorbonne and Heidelberg."

1973–1978: EDWARD ZEGARELLI TAKES OVER

The year after his graduation from Columbia in 1937 Edward Zegarelli joined the faculty as an instructor. He stayed on the faculty and had a

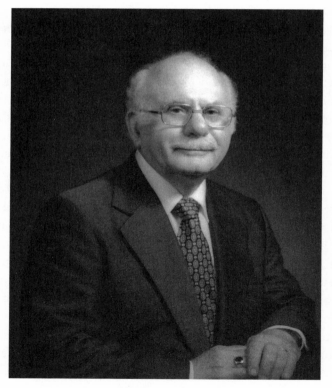

FIGURE 2.12 Dr. Edward Zegarelli (DDS, SDOS 1937) joined the faculty after graduating and served for the next forty-one years on the faculty. He served as dean between 1973 until he retired in 1978. He was an eminent oral pathologist.

distinguished thirty-five-year career at the school. Early in his academic career he began his study and research in a field that would become known as oral medicine. He produced many papers and wrote a definitive textbook on the diagnosis of diseases of the mouth and jaws. He was the director of the Division of Stomatology prior to his appointment as dean. Zegarelli paved the way for two of his sons, David and Peter, at Columbia. All three, Edward and his sons David and Peter, graduated from the University and then completed their DDS education at Columbia, graduating in 1937, 1969, and 1978, respectively. David followed in his father's footsteps as a full-time academic, and Peter taught part time and established a private practice in Tarrytown, New York, his hometown.

Edward Zegarelli became dean in 1973, during his last five years of active service on the Faculty of Dental and Oral Surgery. He was well respected by the full-time faculty and a popular faculty member who was known as an excellent lecturer. Zegarelli was keenly aware of the issues confronting the dental school. He worked to improve the school's finances, continued the initiatives for obtaining state aid, and worked to obtain funds to renovate the facilities. He understood the importance of complying with the recommendations from the last accreditation visit, which called for what he would term a need to improve the "three Fs"—facilities, finances, and full-time faculty. During his tenure he kept in mind that he would need to present a progress report to the Commission on Dental Accreditation (the successor to the CDE) in 1975 and that he had little time to complete some of the work begun under Melvin Moss.

The new dean worked closely with the University president William McGill, the vice president for health sciences Paul Marks and his staff, and the dean of the P&S Donald Tapley. Together they were able to secure New York State capitation aid to help support the cost of educating dental students. To qualify for the state capitation funding, SDOS was required to reserve 70 percent of its entering predoctoral class size for New York State residents. In addition, construction funds from state and federal sources permitted the complete renovation and purchase of new modern dental equipment for the three floors of the school in the Vanderbilt Clinic (floors 7, 8, and 9). A federal grant for that renovation augmented the funds received from the state and provided sufficient funds to complete the renovation, which at that time cost almost

$6 million ($28.5 million in 2014 dollars). This permitted the school to totally gut and modernize these floors, which had been built in 1928. The renovation was completed in 1977, creating a major transformation of facilities and equipment and bringing them to the level of other dental schools in the United States.

There were other important accomplishments under Zegarelli. He understood that he needed to improve the school's standing in the Presbyterian Hospital and the postgraduate programs in the dental school. As a long-time member of the Presbyterian Hospital staff, he strengthened the ties of the school with the hospital, reinstituted a general dental residency program, and normalized the arrangements for operating room privileges. In 1974 he bolstered postgraduate education through the appointment of Irving Naidorf (DDS, SDOS 1941), a clinical professor of endodontics and microbiology, as assistant dean for postgraduate programs.

The University and Medical Center began a new budgeting process for all of the schools in which cost centers were set up that gave each dean control of all of the revenue raised by his school. Each school was to be responsible for covering all of its costs. The dental school conducted its cost study between 1970 and 1975. Stephen Wotman, assistant dean for planning, and Gary Herrmann, MBA and special assistant to the dean, conducted this study. One of the outcomes of the study was to give the dental school control of its clinic revenue. This provided a big incentive for the school to improve the operations of the clinics. Coupled with the improved facilities, the school moved away from department clinics to general clinics in which students were responsible for completing all of the treatment for the patients to whom they were assigned. Under this model, clinic revenue increased while control of expenses improved, and patient care improved thanks to the greater consistency.

All in all, things were looking up. Indeed, the school received its first $1 million gift from the Wood estate in memory of James Benfield, DDS, a long-time faculty member in operative dentistry. When Dean Zegarelli appeared before the Commission on Dental Accreditation on May 5, 1975, to give a progress report on the school, he had a good report to give. The school had made significant progress in solving its problems. In fact, a letter from the commission said just that—but also pointed out that the school still needed to concentrate on improving the ratio of full-time to part-time faculty, finances, and completing the renovation of the clinics. On December 8, 1977, the fully renovated facilities were finally completed and dedicated. With the University president William McGill and the vice president for health sciences Paul Marks in attendance and Julius Richmond, then the U.S. surgeon general, giving a keynote address, the long saga of inadequate facilities ended . . . at least for the moment!

When Dean Zegarelli retired in 1978, a new dean took over, and a new era began.

CHAPTER THREE

1978–2001: The Leap to the Future

Reaching Out

While the School of Dental and Oral Surgery had solved some of its difficult problems during the tenures of Moss and Zegarelli in the late 1960s and through the 1970s, times again were changing dramatically in dental education and on health science campuses by the time the next dean was poised to take over in 1978. A major reassessment of dental education was pushing schools in new directions.[1] While some states without dental schools established new dental schools, seven private universities closed their dental schools. As a result of the closures, existing dental schools were being urged to integrate and better align their missions with those of their medical centers and universities. Curricular advances in hospital dentistry and the need to broaden knowledge, attitudes, and skills of students to meet contemporary needs of the public were stressed.

There were further recommendations regarding expansion of postdoctoral training opportunities in advanced education in general dentistry to better prepare dentists for treating special patient populations such as the physically and mentally challenged. At the same time, society had been drastically altered in the 1960s through the women's movement, Medicaid and Medicare, and affirmative action legislation. All of these changes were affecting educational institutions, including medical and dental schools and their affiliated hospitals. It was a time of great change and Columbia was not exempt.

The Columbia–Presbyterian Medical Center was also going through a series of changes and working to catch up. In 1976, the first new building on the Medical Center campus in more than twenty years opened—the Hammer Health Sciences Building. At the same time, the Presbyterian Hospital was upgrading its antiquated facilities as a temporary fix until a new hospital planned for the mid-1980s could be built. The leadership in the Medical Center expected the SDOS to continue and accelerate the pace of its modernization.

In 1928 Alfred Owre was the last dean to be recruited from outside the school (from the University of Minnesota) until fifty years later, in 1978. That was when the search committee, led by Irwin Mandel, decided it was time to bring in someone who was not on the existing faculty. It ultimately recommended to the vice president for health sciences and the president of the University that Allan J. Formicola[2] become the eleventh dean of the School of Dental and Oral Surgery.

At the time of his appointment, Formicola was thirty-eight years old, young for the position, but rich in requisite experience. After completing all of the prerequisites for dental school at Pennsylvania State University in two years, he was accepted at Georgetown University's School of Dentistry, where he earned his DDS degree and MS degree in periodontics in 1963 and 1965, respectively. He was an early leader in research using radioisotopes to study the development of the supporting apparatus of the teeth. After spending two years in the U.S. Navy, Formicola accepted a full-time teaching position at Georgetown and was soon recruited to the University of Alabama in Birmingham, where he served as an assistant professor of periodontics and investigator in the National Institute of Dental Research–funded Dental Research Center. In 1970 he was appointed as chair of the Department of Periodontics at the College of Medicine and Dentistry of New Jersey, where he subsequently held the positions of associate dean for academic affairs and acting dean before coming to Columbia in 1978.

During Dr. Formicola's deanship, which lasted twenty-three years, several critical changes occurred. First, SDOS successfully shifted from a private, state-related school that received substantial support from the state to a private school that received minor state support. Second, the full-time faculty increased significantly in number and diversity. Third, the mission of the school expanded: patient care and community service became coequal to the education and research missions. Fourth, strategic planning became the means for creating new educational approaches. As a result, SDOS underwent three successful accreditation site visits (1979, 1987, and 1995) by the Commission on Dental Accreditation.

From the very start of his deanship, Formicola had a vision for the school shared by the leadership of the health sciences and the University. In a letter to Paul Marks, the then vice president for health sciences, Formicola presented a blueprint for the dental school designed to meet

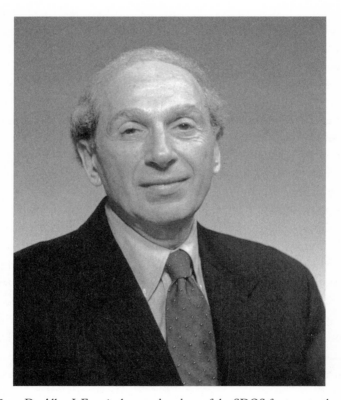

FIGURE 3.1 Dr. Allan J. Formicola served as dean of the SDOS for twenty-three years, from 1978 to 2001. He held positions at the New Jersey Dental School (now the Rutgers School of Dental Medicine), including acting dean prior to moving to Columbia. He also served on the University of Alabama and Georgetown University Dental School faculties.

the challenges of the future. It recommended a thorough review of all programs, growth in the full-time faculty, and new sources of revenue to support the school's mission. Formicola noted that to achieve these goals, assistance from the vice president for health sciences Paul Marks, the dean of the College of Physicians and Surgeons Donald Tapley, and the University president William McGill would be needed. Upon Dr. Formicola's appointment, McGill and Marks approved his overall plan to strengthen the dental school.

THE LEADERSHIP TEAM

During his deanship, Formicola recognized the importance of building a strong administrative group and a team approach to implement changes in the school. Having once served in the capacity of associate dean of academic affairs, he realized that any individual who would serve in that position would be dealing with curricular matters and would function as liaison with P&S. His vision was in harmony with that of the Gies vision and the Columbia tradition of a joint basic science education with the medical school. He selected individuals from the senior faculty to serve as associate deans of academic affairs: first, Dr. Sidney Horowitz in 1979, then Dr. Norman Kahn in 1988, and finally, Dr. Letty Moss-Salentijn in 1992. While the University president nominated Dr. Formicola to be the Robinson Professor of Dentistry, Formicola preferred to nominate the associate deans for academic affairs to hold that title in order to enhance their capacity to help move the school forward.

The administrative team during Formicola's tenure included individuals who understood the Columbia University traditions and culture and were well-versed in the types of changes that would enhance the school's mission. The new dean also recognized the importance of strong financial leadership. Gary Herrmann, a Columbia-educated MBA who was part of the previous administration, was appointed as the assistant dean for administrative affairs and served from 1978 to 1984. Jay Wechsler became assistant dean for financial affairs from 1985 to 1992 and helped to shepherd the school through a financial crisis. His successors in the 1990s, Patricia Long (1992–1997) and Sara Patterson (beginning in 1998), ably managed the school's financial matters.

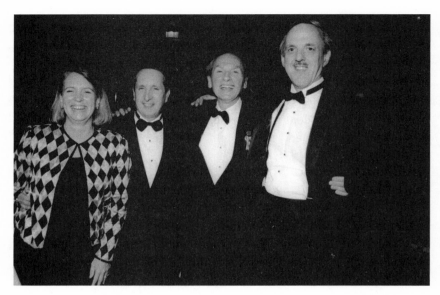

FIGURE 3.2 Three of the four assistant deans for administration and finance who served during Dean Formicola's tenure. Left to right are: Patricia Long, Jay Wechsler, and to the right of Dean Formicola, Gary Herrmann. Not shown is Sara Patterson. They are shown at Dean Formicola's retirement party at the Rotunda of Low Library in September 2001.

These individuals understood the vision for the school's future and were instrumental in managing difficult financial issues while allowing the growth necessary to achieve forward movement in the school.

Other members of the administrative team helped to shape the school under Formicola's leadership. Dr. Irving Naidorf, a respected national leader in the field of endodontics, remained in his previous position of assistant dean for postdoctoral programs until his death. Dr. Martin Davis became assistant dean of student affairs by the end of the 1980s, succeeding Dr. S. Abel Moreinis, who also served up until his untimely death. Dr. Thomas Cangialosi served as assistant dean for student affairs and then became the director of orthodontics and the associate dean for postdoctoral affairs. Later, Dr. Irwin Mandel, who had established the Division of Preventive Dentistry and the Clinical Research Center, became associate dean for research.

PLANNING EFFORTS

SDOS moved forward through a series of productive planning efforts that engaged the faculty and many individuals throughout the University. Each progressive plan enriched the school's education, service, and research missions and deepened its involvement with other schools in the University, the Presbyterian Hospital (as of 1998, the New York Presbyterian Hospital), and eventually the northern Manhattan community.

Reassessment of the school's mission, program goals, and organization took place early in Formicola's deanship. It began with a classic long-range planning process that involved the faculty and evolved to a formal strategic planning initiative. The first annual faculty retreat in 1984 considered future directions for the school. The importance of the outcomes of the planning efforts was emphasized by the attendance of the University president, Michael A. Sovern, and an outside consultant, Dr. Wallace Mann, then the founding and sitting dean of the University of Mississippi Dental School and president of the American Dental Education Association. Both urged the faculty to continue to reshape goals and programs to meet the complex challenges for health sciences schools emerging in the 1980s.

In 1986 a strategic planning effort was implemented through a major grant from the Pew Foundation. It created a two-phased grant program that allowed schools to undertake strategic planning. In phase one, twenty-one schools were funded to rethink their mission, strengths, weaknesses, and opportunities and to plan strategically. In phase two, funds were awarded to implement the changes schools had planned in the first phase, but only six phase two awards were funded. SDOS was successful in obtaining grants from both phases of the program and became one of only six schools in the nation to be awarded a prestigious Pew Foundation grant of $1.1 million to plan and implement strategic change. The Pew grant enabled the school to deal with financial issues during difficult times while making important program advances.

These planning efforts guided the school into a twenty-year period of growth and renewal. However, SDOS still needed to deal with new financial challenges, as a major and abrupt shift occurred in New York State support.

FINANCES: THE SCHOOL OF DENTAL AND ORAL SURGERY SHIFTS FROM A PRIVATE, STATE-RELATED SCHOOL TO A PRIVATE SCHOOL

During his deanship, Formicola had to work within the University budgetary process, which required schools to cover the cost of their operations and find funds for advancement. The growth he envisioned in the school's mission and programs necessitated new funds over and above the school's base budget. However, the last two decades of the twentieth century proved to be challenging for dental schools across the country. The closure of seven private dental schools in the 1980s and early 1990s raised the question of the financial viability of all dental schools, especially the remaining private dental schools, including Columbia. At Columbia, a loss of federal and state capitation support for the dental school during the late 1980s signaled the end of two decades of governmental interest in expanding the dental workforce. The reduction of state aid alone reduced the dental school's outside support by 24 percent, a difficult and challenging situation. During this period, these national and local issues weighed heavily on SDOS, requiring the development of plans that were true to the culture and traditions of Columbia but also aggressive and forward thinking.

Growth in resources on which to base program renewal was essential. Upon arrival at the school in 1978, Dr. Formicola embraced a somewhat controversial Coopers and Lybrand consultant report that called for the modernization of systems in the clinic. It called for a shift from operating the clinics as teaching clinics oriented toward student needs, which were inefficient providers of patient care, to more efficiently operated clinics that were more oriented toward patient needs. The University had shifted to a responsibility budgeting system under which clinic revenue was to be retained by the dental school and used as an important source of new funds on which to base program improvements. Computer systems to manage the clinic and academic programs were an essential resource.

One of the first initiatives Formicola undertook was an application for a federal grant then available to strengthen the school's finances. Within the first six months of his deanship, the school received $500,000 from a government financial distress grant. This first grant enabled the school to catch up with other dental schools in the country in the use of technology in both education and management. The funds enabled the school to enter the digital era. SDOS built its first computer system to manage the billing in the dental clinic. Funds were also used to invest in educational technology to improve the efficiency of the faculty. In the early 1980s an audiovisual unit was created by hiring an audiovisual expert, Douglas McAndrew. Then, under the leadership of Dr. John Zimmerman, one of the early leaders in what was then the new field of dental informatics, the school expanded its computer-based programs in the 1990s. By the late 1990s the audiovisual-dental informatics program had grown into the health sciences unit for the Columbia University Center for New Media, Teaching and Learning supporting all four health sciences schools—the dental school and the schools of medicine, public health, and nursing—to improve pedagogy. This media center continues to help the faculty develop and employ multimedia approaches in their courses, including computer-based online systems.

A Loss of New York State Funding

The school's financial resources, which were much improved by the end of the 1970s, continued to grow until the late 1980s, when financial problems hit again. In the early 1980s, with the strong advocacy of Dean Formicola and the assistance of Dr. William Polf, the health sciences vice president for government and community affairs, a second source of state revenue, the dental clinic subsidy program, was added. By the 1988–1989 year, approximately 25 percent of the school's revenue was from federal/state sources, the majority of which was from New York State through the capitation and dental clinic subsidy programs. Hence, the school became classified as a private, state-related school in recognition of this partnership and reserved 70 percent of the entering predoctoral seats for New York State residents as a condition of receiving the capitation award.

Support from New York State ended during the 1988 and 1989 budget years, years in which the state was experiencing budget shortfalls. The state ended the capitation program for the thirteen private medical schools in New York and the two private dental schools at Columbia University and New York University. Congress had previously ended the federal capitation program as well. To add insult to injury, New York State reduced the dental clinic subsidy program to Columbia and New York University. Columbia's award decreased from $1.2 million per year to slightly less than $500,000. The school lost almost 25 percent of its revenue in two budget years. Many predicted it would not be able to recover from this severe financial blow over such a short period of time. They were wrong.

Digging Out of the Financial Hole

The school reached financial solvency thanks to a multipronged approach. Several initiatives led to this: an increase in income from patient care, other new fund-raising efforts, and judicious reductions in spending. As a result of the strategic planning process, the school had adopted a broader vision for the patient care mission to become more service oriented and productive. Evening clinic hours to service those residents of northern Manhattan who worked, summer clinic sessions, and greater efficiency in providing care all helped to alleviate the funding crisis brought on by the abrupt loss of federal and state support.

The student clinical programs advanced through a comprehensive patient care program and a quality assurance program. These were designed so that care provided in the student clinics was more efficient than before, and clinic revenue improved as a result. Patient surveys showed that patient satisfaction improved as well. Providers grew beyond students to include licensed dentists, both faculty and fellows, an idea originally espoused by Alfred Owre and later followed by many other dental schools. Thus, under the leadership of the dean of clinical affairs, a new position established with the appointment of Dr. Ennio Uccelani from 1979 to 1985 and, subsequently, Dr. Ronnie Myers beginning in 1986, patient care revenue grew beyond expectations. It exploded 44 percent between the 1984–1985 year and the 1988–1989 year (the year of the cutback of state support) and grew from $1.3 million to $3 million. Indeed, there was a doubling in the number of patient visits provided in the on-site clinical programs from 40,000 to 80,000 by 1996–1997.

Revenue was also enhanced through a faculty practice dental insurance plan. The University president, Michael Sovern, asked Formicola to develop a plan to provide dental coverage for the University faculty, because the health plan did not provide dental coverage. Many faculty members on the Morningside campus were also calling for such a plan. In response, the school developed the Columbia Dental Plan, designed specifically to treat University faculty. Begun in 1993 under the direction of Dr. Stephen Marshall, the Columbia Dental Plan has grown over the years, and in 2014 covered more than 10,000 Columbia University employees. They now receive their dental care from the full-time dental school faculty in the faculty practice plan or from part-time faculty in their private offices in 221 practitioner locations. A dental plan was also developed to cover all of the University students on the Morningside campus. The faculty practice plan permitted the school to improve the salary structure for full-time faculty, which was essential to recruit new faculty and to relieve the school's base budget of having to provide all of the salary support for faculty. By 1988–1989 patient care revenue was approximately 19 percent of all revenue helping to plug the gap from the reduction of state aid.

A newly established annual fund and a capital campaign were established, further helping to cushion the blow of the loss of federal and state aid and fueling many of the changes. The alumni association worked closely with Dr. Irving Naidorf to create a new category of annual giving for major donors called the 1852 Society. (The name referred to the dental school chartered in 1852 in Syracuse, New York, a charter inherited by the College of Dental and Oral Surgery, the school that Columbia absorbed into its Dental School. See Chapter 1 and Appendix 2 for more on this history.) In addition to annual giving campaigns, two successive five-year capital fund-raising campaigns begun in the mid-1980s raised $15 million, of which approximately $10 million was spent to reconstruct the preclinical and clinical facilities and to renovate more than 6,000 square feet of new space assigned to the school on the Presbyterian Hospital 7 East floor in the building at 168th Street. The fund-raising activities also increased the number of the school's endowed professorships from two (Robinson and Benefield) to five (with the addition of Zegarelli, Guttman, and Richter). This growth in resources was unprecedented in the school's history and made programs of renewal possible. These fund-raising efforts, along with corporate giving and private grants, grew to be 6 percent of the budget.

But this was still not enough to deal with the loss of federal and state support. It was also essential to reduce spending. The dean and division directors were able to agree on a cutback plan that preserved the major advances already achieved and to continue the program of renewal. The plan entailed reducing a significant number of the two-day-per-week paid part-time faculty positions, the numbers of which had grown significantly over the 1980s. Most of these faculty members understood that they could fall back on their private practices to replace this income. Many remained as one-day volunteer faculty members.

Finally, the medical school loaned the dental school $600,000 to replace a portion of the state aid lost. The dean made the case to the vice president for health sciences and dean of the College of Physicians and Surgeons, Dr. Herbert Pardes, that cutting any further would greatly reduce the quality of the school and curtail forward progress. The vice president concurred. The school paid back the loan over the next several years.

All of these efforts paid off. Even with the loss of state funding, school revenue grew significantly over the twenty-year period from $10.5 million in 1984–1985 to $32.1 million by the year 2000. Early in the development of the revenue base for the school in the late 1970s through the 1980s, New York State had become one of the most important sources of revenue; by the 1990s this situation had changed. The school was able to shift its resource base as described above after the state and federal funding ended, which was a surprise to many.

During the 1990s, then, due to good planning and a strenuous effort by the faculty and staff, the school was able to recover from the financial setback from the loss of federal and state funding. By the end of the 1990s, the school had only 2 percent of its budget from state support and was once again a private school. The school no longer had to reserve 70 percent of its seats for New York State residents and recruited nationally. During the 1990s approximately 20 percent of the students were from New York State, and the school had become more national and international in scope. In the 2000–2001 year, for example, seventeen first-year students were from New York, twenty-five from California, six from New Jersey, and the remainder of the class was from thirteen other states across the nation, with eight students coming from foreign countries.

FACULTY TURNOVER AND ADDITIONAL FACULTY
SPUR GROWTH

At the beginning of Formicola's deanship in 1978, the leadership of the full-time faculty was composed mainly of tenured senior rank individuals, all of whom were Columbia graduates from the 1940s. To meet the challenges of the times, these faculty members recognized the need for a shift and fully participated in the development of programs of improvement. These individuals included Drs. Irwin Mandel, Robert Gottsegen, Joseph Leavitt, John Lucca, Edward Cain, Nicholas DiSalvo, Ennio Uccelani, Solon (Art) Ellison, and Irving Naidorf, with the latter serving as assistant dean for postdoctoral programs.

These faculty recognized the need to recruit and develop the junior faculty ranks, especially those with diverse backgrounds. There were almost no junior faculty members, because few assistant professors had been added to the full-time faculty during the 1970s. During the late 1980s and early 1990s, these senior professors all retired, but during their tenures they worked closely with the dean and the associate deans for academic affairs to recruit new faculty members and make the necessary changes to strengthen the school.

The growth in the clinical faculty was assisted by alterations in the tenure rules in the 1970s. The University approved the creation at the health sciences of an additional non-tenure track, the clinical professor track. The clinical professor track was intended to assist the medical and dental school's recruitment of full-time faculty whose main responsibilities would be patient care and teaching. SDOS vigorously took advantage of the clinical professor's track to expand the clinical faculty. By 1988 the full-time faculty had grown from twenty-nine to fifty-four as twenty-five new full-time faculty members of all ranks had been recruited, including two oral and maxillofacial surgeons, and three dentists with PhDs. By 1995 the school had largely rebuilt the junior ranks.

As a result of the process of appointing a formal search committee for each available position, the full-time faculty grew in diversity as well as in number. For example, of the twenty-five full-time assistant professors in place in 1995, eleven were women, three held PhDs, two held both the DDS and MD degrees, four held the DDS and MPH degrees, and twelve had specialty training. Their degrees were earned at thirteen universities, including such renowned institutions as Harvard and the University of North Carolina. By the turn of the millennium, SDOS had the highest percent of African American faculty of all dental schools in the nation with the exception of Howard and Meharry. In a ripple effect, their arrival helped the school to improve the diversity of the student body.

The school's leadership continued to evolve as well. New faculty had arrived in the 1980s to replace and expand upon the large wave of retirees who had originally joined the faculty in the 1940s and 1950s. During the 1990s much of the school's new leadership arose from this expansion of the faculty. By the year 2000 the full-time faculty had grown to seventy-five positions practicing on-site in the Vanderbilt Clinic and off-site at facilities on the University's Morningside Heights campus, at the Presbyterian Hospital's East Sixtieth Street facility, and four community health centers in the Washington Heights and Harlem communities.

Without doubt, one of the major strengths for Columbia was access to world-class clinicians in the New York metropolitan area. Columbia's

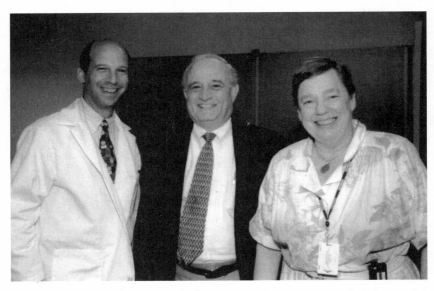

FIGURE 3.3 Dr. John Scarola (SDOS 1960), a part-time volunteer faculty member, is congratulated by Drs. Ron Myers and Letty Moss Salentijn after receiving the Allan J. Formicola Teaching Award.

faculty continued to be enriched by the more than 100 part-time voluntary faculty members and other faculty members appointed at the twenty-three affiliated hospitals and community centers to which students and residents rotated. They continued to bring the perspective of the real-world challenges of private practice into teaching and provided opportunities for the students to learn the complexities of treating the most vulnerable individuals within the dental clinics of the metropolitan hospitals and community centers of New York City.

The increase in faculty permitted major program advances, including an expansion in the research programs, renewal of the predoctoral curriculum, enlargement of the postdoctoral and hospital-based programs, and an extension of the mission to address social issues impacting the profession and segments of the public in the oral health-care arena.

GROWTH IN RESEARCH EFFORTS

Back in 1926 the report by SDOS founder William Gies urged dental schools to encourage the growth of a full-time faculty, in part to stimulate investigations in the field of dental medicine. A review of the publications over the last twenty years (1980–2001) of Formicola's tenure demonstrated the wide interest of the faculty in areas such as oral biology, pathology, systemic-oral disease interactions, and dental materials. Faculty publications in journals ranged from ninety-five in the 1985–1986 year to sixty-five in the 1990–1991 year and 112 in the 2000–2001 year—a respectable effort given the small size of the faculty.

However, during the last two decades of the twentieth century, the school also recognized that it needed to recruit a critical mass of full-time faculty able to conduct research at a high level. This was vital to compete effectively with the top ten dental schools in the nation for external research funding from the National Institute of Dental and Craniofacial Research (NIDCR).

SDOS had many barriers to overcome in achieving this goal, especially a paucity of seed funds for pilot projects, limited research laboratory facilities, and a basic science faculty attached to the medical school. The dean recognized the school would have to compete with well-funded state schools, five of which had attracted dental institutes funded by the

National Institutes of Health in the 1960s. Undaunted by these barriers, SDOS looked to its strengths and recognized that the close relationship between the faculties in the health sciences schools presented opportunities. However, certain infrastructure issues required attention in order to fuel the development of a research program at a level that would permit SDOS to become a research-intense dental school.

First, all of the postdoctoral training programs were certificate programs. So there were no graduate-level students enrolled at the school, and few schools succeed in research without the interaction between graduate students and faculty. Second, the school lacked laboratory space. And third, SDOS would need to recruit new research leadership.

To address the first problem, in the early 1980s, under the leadership of Dr. S. Arthur Ellison, SDOS added an optional master of arts program through the Graduate School of Arts and Sciences for those postdoctoral certificate students enrolled in the specialty programs. This provided a cadre of graduate students who wished to pursue a serious research investigation along with their clinical training.

To address the second problem, in 1988 the school obtained a 2,300 square foot block of new space on Presbyterian Hospital 7 Center. Dr. Irwin Mandel led the establishment of the Center for Clinical Research in Dentistry. Mandel, a 1945 SDOS graduate, joined the faculty in 1946 as a research assistant and became a full-time member of the faculty by 1968. He was elected president of the American Association of Dental Research in 1981 and became the first recipient of the American Dental Association Gold Medal for Excellence in Dental Research in 1985. Irwin Mandel was a mentor for a number of SDOS students and others who later pursued successful research careers. Mandel's laboratory was always a hub of activity for students and junior faculty interested in research. He was also honored for his outstanding efforts in mentoring by being awarded the first American Association of Dental Research Distinguished Mentoring Award in 2010. Mandel was the type of full-time faculty member that Gies envisioned in dental schools. He established ties with researchers in the Medical Center, specifically in ophthalmology and dermatology. His studies on salivary chemistry helped in the diagnosis of Sjogren's syndrome. Many of his studies on saliva and dental caries were landmark in scope.

Mandel was world renowned not only for his research and leadership accomplishments but also for his wit and wisdom, which kept audiences always looking forward to one of his presentations. Ernest Newbrun, professor emeritus at the University of California, San Francisco, dubbed him an "inveterate punster" and compiled a pamphlet called *Quotations from Chairman Mandel*, which collected many of Mandel's witty comments made at his talks or found in his writings. The one quotation that Mandel was most known for is titled "Creation," which poked fun at researchers: "When God created Man, he gave him blood for hematologists to study, sweat for dermatologists to study, tears for ophthalmologists to study, urine for urologists to study, gingival fluid for periodontologists to study and saliva for oral biologists to study."

The establishment of the clinical research center provided the initial momentum to expand the school's research agenda. Later, in the early 1990s, the school received 6,000 square feet of additional expansion space on Presbyterian Hospital 7 East in which additional laboratories were constructed for the Division of Periodontics. Even though these research facilities were meager in comparison to those of other dental schools, they were sufficient to stimulate the buildup of a critical mass of research faculty.

Keeping in mind the need to collaborate with faculty in the medical and public health schools, the two schools with which SDOS has joint education programs, the research program took shape around two programmatic areas. The first studied the interrelationship of oral infection, oral inflammation, and systemic disease. This research was stimulated and led by Dr. Ira Lamster, who was recruited in 1988 as director of the Division of Periodontics. The second area of investigation included the oral health needs of underserved population groups. It was led by Dr. Donald Sadowsky, who was recruited to redevelop the Division of Community Health.

Both program areas attracted significant new funds from the NIH. Studies were begun on HIV infection and dentistry by Dr. Irwin Mandel (salivary component), Dr. Ira Lamster (onset of periodontal infections), and Dr. Donald Sadowsky (dental management of HIV-positive patients). The systemic–oral disease interactions research grew as additional researchers, such as Dr. Panos Papapanou, were recruited by Dr. Lamster. Their collaborations included work on the implications of periodontal infections on diabetes with Drs. Evanthia Lalla in periodontics and Ann Marie Schmidt in the Department of Medicine, and studies on the relationship of stroke and periodontal disease with Stephen Engebretson in periodontics, Ralph Sacco in neurology, and Moise Desvarieux in the School of Public Health. Dr. Lamster was able to understand that investigators in the Department of Medicine, the Neurologic Institute, and the School of Public Health would be eager to collaborate with investigators in the dental school when the studies were scientifically important. By the late 1990s these investigations were competitive enough to qualify for funding from the National Institute of Dental and Craniofacial Research.

Adding to this renewed research program in the divisions were schoolwide projects in the development of the public service mission of the dental school. The community effort yielded research information that developed a keener understanding of the epidemiology of dental caries in African Americans and Hispanics (led by Dr. Dennis Mitchell and Dr. David Albert in community health with Dr. Sally Findley and Luisa Borrell in the School of Public Health) and the relationship of oral infection to preterm and low-birth-weight babies (led by Dr. Panos Papapanou, director of periodontics, and Dr. Dennis Mitchell). Research advanced over the years into studies of multidisciplinary systems approaches to oral health; the impact of culture, insurance coverage, and dental fear on oral health; and geriatric dentistry. Twenty-five peer-reviewed publications have resulted so far from the development of the Community DentCare program in addition to its important contribution to providing access to care for northern Manhattan residents and sites for the education of predoctoral and postdoctoral students.

This major growth in the research program is evident when reviewing outside research support from government and nongovernmental sources. It grew from around $1 million in 1984 to approximately $2.2 million in 1992 and to nearly $3.5 million in the 2000–2001 year.

RENEWAL OF THE PREDOCTORAL CURRICULUM

From the inception of the Columbia School of Dental and Oral Surgery curriculum, its hallmark has been the strong biomedical course work offered as joint instruction to both medical and dental students. But by the mid-1980s, the curriculum had become overcrowded with dental courses in the first two years. This made it difficult for students to succeed in the basic science courses at the same level as the medical students. In an important meeting of Dean Formicola with the associate dean for academic affairs, Norman Kahn, and the department chairs of the basic science departments, it was agreed that the dental school would reduce the dental course load in the first two years so that the students could better concentrate on the basic science courses. Furthermore, the clinical curriculum was not keeping pace with contemporary curricula in schools throughout the nation. Therefore, four overarching revisions were planned and put into place. They were:

1. decompression of course content in the first two years to permit students more time to study and assimilate the basic sciences;
2. a medical core of course work to enhance students' abilities to monitor patients' overall health;
3. reorganization of the third- and fourth-year clinical programs; and
4. electives, called areas of concentration, in the third and fourth years to give students an opportunity to explore special interests.

The reorganization of the curriculum took place between 1988 and 1995. The strategic planning process supported by the Pew Foundation in the mid-1980s allowed the rethinking of the DDS curriculum. It engaged the entire faculty through retreats and various planning committees. Norman Kahn played a leadership role in the reorganization of the curriculum. Stephen Marshall (DDS, State University of New York, Buffalo 1986, and MPH, Columbia 1989) was hired to manage the strategic planning process.

Decompression of Courses to Permit Reemphasis of the Basic Science Education

There was general agreement among the faculty that a major redesign of the curriculum was required to permit students to gain the needed time in the first two years to perform well in the basic science course work. The preclinical course load and contact hours were reduced in the first two years so that students could absorb the strong basic science education. This allowed the dental students to be on par with the medical students in performance. This was contrary to most of the other dental schools in the nation, which had decreased the basic science course content to permit a heavier course load of preclinical and clinical courses in the first two years. Columbia, along with the schools of dental medicine at Harvard University, University of Connecticut, and SUNY Stony Brook were at the time (and remain) the only four dental schools in the nation to still subscribe to joint basic science courses for medical and dental students. Columbia was fortunate to have been developed around close relationships with the medical school. The faculty recognized this as an important strength of the school that had to be preserved.

A Medical Core of Instruction

A two-year planning effort by an ad hoc committee to reexamine the curriculum under the leadership of Dr. Nicholas Di Salvo recognized the importance of dental students taking a medical core, which included the second-year medical school pathophysiology course followed by a course in physical diagnosis. This was recommended for future dentists to be able to better manage the care of the growing number of older individuals in the United States and others with significant medical histories being kept alive by advances in medical science.

The pathophysiology course, offered by the Department of Medicine, was opened to the dental students, as the chair of that department,

Dr. Robert Glickman, recognized the need for the dental students to have such a course. The Division of Oral and Maxillofacial Surgery took on the responsibility to follow up the lecture program with small-group teaching and a physical diagnosis course. A two-week rotation to hospitals was the culmination of the medical core and provided students with experience in working with oral surgery residents on patient histories and diagnosis.

A survey of the class of 1993, at the end of their third year, showed that 76 percent of the class rated the medical core training as very important to their overall education. Students indicated that half of their patients presented with significant medical histories requiring such knowledge. Many postdoctoral and hospital training directors are pleased with Columbia graduates in relation to graduates from other schools because of their strong understanding of the importance of the patient's medical history and their knowledge of basic science.

Reorganizing the Third- and Fourth-Year Clinical Program

Further, the clinical education in the third and fourth years was reorganized to make the students' transition into providing patient care less stressful and to emphasize the behavioral and social sciences in patient management. The ad hoc curriculum committee reconceptualized the clinical curriculum to create a more gradual introduction into patient care for the third-year students.[4] Instead of assigning patients to students and expecting the students to perform a full range of clinical procedures at the beginning of the third year, which in reality the students were not prepared to do, the new curriculum emphasized the need for students to gain the building blocks for comprehensive care by the end of the third year. Basic experience in diagnosis and treatment planning and simple clinical procedures, with a more gradual introduction to patient care, became the design for the third-year clinic. A monthlong rotation to a hospital on an oral surgical service rounded out the third-year experience.

The postdoctoral fellows in general dentistry assisted the third-year students through their introductory patient care year. Rather than adhering to the traditional approach of counting the number of procedures a student performs to determine whether a student is ready to

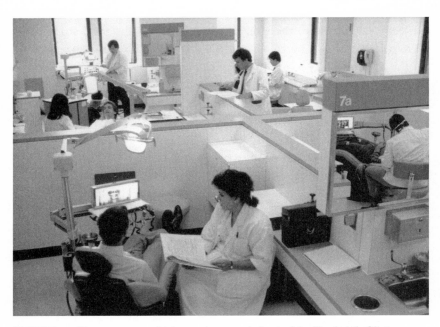

FIGURE 3.4 The treatment cubicles on the seventh floor of the Vanderbilt Clinic were reconstructed in the late 1970s. This floor was designated for fourth-year students treating their comprehensive-care patients. This photograph of the SDOS dental clinic was taken around 1992.

move up to fourth-year status, the faculty, under the leadership of Drs. Richard Lichtenthal and Laureen Zubiaurre Bitzer, developed an evaluation system to determine whether students had achieved competence in diagnosis, treatment planning, and basic clinical procedures through a series of tests. Upon completion of this testing, students were then given greater patient care responsibility beginning in the summer after third year and moved along in developing their diagnostic, treatment planning, and clinical skills.

The fourth year was designed to include a one-day-per-week rotation to a hospital, where the students obtained more and varied clinical experience. In a major departure from the traditional dental school requirements, the faculty, under the leadership of Drs. Richard Lichtenthal and Vicky Evangelides, no longer judged students ready for graduation based on the number of clinical procedures accomplished, instead using a system that determined how well the students managed the entire care for a group of patients they were assigned to treat.[5] Dr. Evangelides stressed the importance of patients receiving comprehensive care, and students were held responsible for all of the care of their patients, even if they had to refer them for specialty care. Group discussion of cases became an important component of the learning environment under Dr. Evangelides's guidance and helped in the evaluation of students' progress. This system of evaluation required the faculty to become more sophisticated in its assessment process and to work more closely with students on providing patient care.

To implement the fourth-year clinical curriculum and broaden students' education in the behavioral and social sciences, a new section, the Comprehensive Care Section, was organized in the 1983–1984 year. Behavioral management of the patient and an understanding of cultural factors had been underemphasized in the curriculum. Several formally independent divisions (behavioral science, community health, practice management, preventive dentistry, and pediatric dentistry) with faculty able to enrich this portion of the curriculum formed this new section. Under the leadership of Dr. Martin Davis (SDOS 1974), for a period of six years this section enriched the curriculum with course work in the domain of the behavioral sciences and public health with the assistance of Dr. Lynn Tepper, a behavioral scientist, and with the addition of faculty such as Dr. David Albert, who held both DDS and MPH degrees.

The Comprehensive Care Section brought innovation to the clinical curriculum by teaching communication skills, emphasizing the importance of obtaining a social and cultural patient history, developing geriatric course work, and demonstrating that patient care is more than performing clinical procedures. The fourth-year clinical program, the senior practice program, was designed to include weekly patient care seminars for students to discuss and reflect on the cases they were treating with their faculty mentors. Under Dr. Davis's leadership, the section gave credibility to the sociomedical and behavioral aspects of dental education. Although the divisions under the Comprehensive Care Section became reorganized once again in the 1990s, the curriculum innovation this section was responsible for encouraging continued.

Another important subject was added to the curriculum that set the pace for similar courses in schools throughout New York and the rest of the nation. Dr. Robert Miner (SDOS 1967), a longtime volunteer faculty member, created a professional ethics course in the curriculum through actual case studies collected by volunteer faculty. The New York Academy of Dentistry organized this effort with Dr. Miner. Robert Miner has long ties to Columbia through his father, Dwight Carroll Miner (CC 1926, PhD 1940), who was a well-known history professor at the University. Interestingly, the elder Miner edited the University's Bicentennial History of Columbia University published between 1954 and 1957.

Electives and the Area of Concentration Program

The fourth curriculum change stimulated by the strategic planning effort and the ad hoc curriculum committee was the design of two years of electives organized around an area of concentration. The notion behind this curricular advance was to permit each student to study an area of interest beyond the required curriculum. Dr. Marlene Klyvert organized and managed the program and provided students with a thorough orientation. Then, all students selected an area of concentration from several tracks ranging from research to beyond-the-core course work in the dental specialties and from tracks in research, veterinary dentistry, and community dentistry to cross-registering for degree programs in public health and business. Students were able to cross-register for courses on the Morningside campus, and many took advantage of this option.

The area of concentration program was modeled on a previous program of the same name that was discontinued due to a ruling disallowing it by the Commission on Dental Accreditation. Despite their similarities, there were two major differences between the two programs. The first difference was that the previous program combined the fourth year of dental school and the first year of postdoctoral training in the dental specialties, not joint degrees with other schools. The second difference was that the previous program was open to only the top 10 percent of students, whereas its successor program was open to and required of all students, and encouraged joint degrees with other schools. Even in the early years of SDOS under Dean Owre, it was recognized that electives should be available to students, and this program fulfilled that vision.

The joint degree opportunities made possible through the area of concentration program were attractive options for students. Twenty-five students were awarded the MPH/DDS degree and several students earned the DDS/MBA degree during the last decade of the twentieth century and the first decade of the twenty-first. Two graduates who selected these options as students are profiled here. Mayra Suero-Wade completed the DDS/MPH program, and Saleem Josephs completed the requirements for three degrees—a DDS, an MPH, and an MBA—in five years!

ALUMNI VOICES: MAYRA SUERO-WADE

Mayra Suero-Wade, DDS, MPH, is practicing in New York City and New Jersey and provides care to underserved children. She is a part-time associate professor of dentistry at the College of Dental Medicine. Suero-Wade was raised in the Dominican Republic and came to America with her family at age twelve. The family lived in Washington Heights. Mayra attended New York University on a full scholarship, earning a bachelor of arts degree in 1982.

She dreamed of becoming a dentist who would make a difference in the lives of people who lacked proper dental care. She says, "I applied to four dental schools and was accepted to Columbia, my number 1 choice! I wanted to stay in New York City, the greatest city in the world, for my dental school education and attend Columbia, the best dental school."

She says her particular strengths were in patient care and making dentures. She had a natural ability to visualize what the final denture product should look like, and as a result became the go-to student for helping her peers set up teeth for dentures. She especially loved the last two years of dental school, because that was when she "started taking care of the dental needs of my patients. Relating to them and providing them the dental relief and care they needed was wonderful." She looked up to Dean Formicola as a mentor, saying, "He was highly respected for his consistency, fairness and strength. Plus, he was very approachable. My other mentor was Dr. Albert Thompson."

Mayra graduated in 1988 with dual degrees, the DDS and the MPH, which enabled her to branch out into many areas: private practice, public health, business enterprise, consulting, education, and philanthropy. "Doing the combined degree program and getting my Master of Public Health degree at Columbia opened the door for me to develop my portable dental program named Dentistry In Motion." More than twenty years ago Dr. Suero-Wade made dental care available to agencies that provide health services to children in foster care. At that time, she discovered that only 17 percent of children in foster care were under the care of a dentist. Dr. Suero-Wade purchased portable dental equipment and used her master's in public health experience to develop an in-house dental care program to serve all of the children at New York Foundling. As a result, the dental compliance rate soared above 80 percent in six months.

Not surprisingly, Suero-Wade has won a number of awards and citations from New York City, New York State, New Jersey, and other jurisdictions, including an honorary doctorate degree of humane letters from Felician College. She says, "I believe that Columbia University is a brand that is recognized and respected worldwide. The educational opportunities at Columbia are endless, I have returned time and time again for continuing education courses and feel connected to cutting-edge dental techniques that help me keep up with advances in the profession. My Columbia education has truly been a blessing!"

ALUMNI VOICES: SALEEM JOSEPHS AND FAMILY

Saleem Josephs, his wife Katayoun (Kat) Yaraghi-Josephs, and his two brothers, Philip and Elias, all took advantage of the joint programs through the area of concentration program and cross-registration with the Mailman School of Public Health and the Columbia Business School. It is quite a record and unique in the history of the college.

In 2006 Saleem completed three degrees in five years, the DDS, the MPH, and the MBA, which is no easy task; Katayoun and Philip completed both the DDS and MPH degrees in 2005 and 2008, respectively. Elias earned the DDS and MBA degrees in 2010.

After graduation Saleem spent almost a decade in the financial world in health-care investment banking, first at Bear Stearns Companies and then at Bank of America Merrill Lynch. Dr. Josephs recently returned to the dental field, and he and his wife have brought a "Midtown"-type dental practice to "Uptown" in Washington Heights. The goal of the practice is to provide a full range of treatment options, including implants, to improve access to quality care for underserved ethnic minority communities not far from his alma mater. He says, "This venture is the culmination of all three disciplines pursued while at Columbia."

Organizing practices where the payer mix contains a high percentage of patients covered by Medicaid has proven difficult. However, with Saleem's education at Columbia and experience in the financial world, the Washington Heights practice is functioning well. They are moving to replicate and scale the model elsewhere this year. Brothers Philip and Elias have continued on to postdoctoral training after completing their studies at Columbia. Philip completed the periodontic postdoctoral program at the University of California, Los Angeles, and in 2015 graduated from the orthodontic postdoctoral program at the University of Pennsylvania. Elias continued on to the pediatric dentistry postdoctoral program at Lutheran Hospital in Brooklyn. He is now in private practice in Naples, Florida. The Josephs brothers all came to Columbia from their home in Jamaica.

The curricular revisions and the redesign of the clinical curriculum, now called the "step plan curriculum design" (not to be confused with the STEP program described later in this chapter),[6] continued to attract a well-qualified DDS student body. In fact, the admissions office noted that the shift to a national recruitment process and the new curriculum were responsible for the enrollment of the most prepared classes as measured by the Dental Aptitude Test. The mean DAT academic average for the class enrolling in 2000, for example, placed them in the 95th percentile of all applicants nationwide. During this period of time, the number of women enrolled grew to become 40 percent of the entering students in 1997–1998, up from less than 10 percent in the early 1980s.

POSTDOCTORAL AND HOSPITAL RESIDENCY PROGRAMS

The school's postdoctoral education and hospital residency programs were also greatly strengthened and expanded during this time. In 1978 the school sponsored the well-recognized and respected two-year certificate postdoctoral specialty programs in periodontics, endodontics, pediatric dentistry, and orthodontics. In 1984–1985 under the strong urging of the director of the Division of Prosthodontics, Dr. John Lucca, the two-year postdoctoral specialty program in prosthodontics was reactivated. Subsequent directors, Drs. James Schweigert and Robert Wright, continued to build the prosthodontic postgraduate program into one that included an optional maxillofacial prosthodontic residency year in collaboration with the Bronx Veterans Administration Hospital. The postdoctoral specialty programs in these four disciplines continued to flourish with the addition of a master of arts degree option to the certificate program. The programs attracted a highly competitive group of national and international students. In the 1996–1997 year, for example, there were fifty students enrolled in the four programs, including students from Greece, Italy, Israel, France, Brazil, Korea, Taiwan, and the Virgin Islands.

ORAL AND MAXILLOFACIAL SURGERY AND HOSPITAL DENTISTRY

Early in Formicola's tenure as dean, it was decided that the first area of major growth in the school would be to build the hospital-based programs. In the mid-1970s Dean Zegarelli had reinstituted a one-year hospital residency program in general dentistry sponsored by the Presbyterian Hospital. He also had secured important new privileges to use the Presbyterian Hospital's operating room. Subsequently, Dean Formicola sought to build on this opening with the hospital and deepened the relationship by working with the president of the hospital, Dr. Felix De Martini. In a key meeting arranged by the hospital president, Dean Formicola proposed to the chair of the Department of Surgery, Dr. Keith Reemsma, Dr. Thomas Krizek, the head of plastic surgery, and the chair of otolaryngology, Dr. Maxwell Abramson, to recruit a full-time director of the Division of Oral Surgery and Chief of the Hospital Dental Service. It was understood that to recruit the strongest individual a new hospital-sponsored residency program in oral and maxillofacial surgery would be required. This was an important meeting because in an earlier era (the 1950s and 1960s), there had been constant disagreements between the head and neck surgeons and the oral surgery program with the result being a termination of the latter's residency program. By gaining the agreement of these individuals and including them in the search process, Formicola was able to secure the necessary hospital support for the development of a major new effort in hospital dentistry.

In the 1970s, the school's Division of Oral Surgery had been headed by two very able and dedicated part-time faculty oral surgeons, Drs. George Minervini and Louis Mandel. However, the programs under their direction were limited to DDS students. Irwin Mandel headed the search committee to recruit a full-time oral surgeon. The school appointed Steven Roser (DMD, Harvard 1968), who had also completed the Harvard combined MD–oral and maxillofacial surgery program in 1972. By 1982 Dr. Roser had initiated the combined MD–oral and maxillofacial surgery residency program at the Presbyterian

ALUMNI VOICES: CHRISTOPHER BONACCI

When SDOS decided to rebuild its Presbyterian Hospital dental programs in the 1970s and the 1980s, the school wanted a strong oral and maxillofacial surgery residency program combined with an MD degree. Such a program would need to enroll highly motivated and well-prepared residents. Christopher Bonacci is one of those students who completed ten years at SDOS and P&S for that training. Bonacci credits his success to Dr. Stephen Roser, the director of the oral and maxillofacial surgery residency program and the founder of the program at SDOS, and Dr. Martin Davis, dean of students, who Bonacci recalls, "Both believed in me and saw something in me that led me into my area of specialization." Without their support, he continues, "my life would be very different than it is today." He fondly remembers both Drs. Lou Mandel and Harold Baurmash—two longtime faculty members in oral surgery—for motivating him to expect nothing but outstanding outcomes in his treatment of patients.

Dr. Bonacci is in private practice in Vienna, Virginia. About his overall experience at Columbia he said: "I remain grateful to Columbia for shaping me and molding me into the professional that I am today. I regularly look back at the great memories I made at 168th Street and Broadway over a ten-year period of time that passed far too quickly. In reflection, I am truly in awe of the people I had a chance to work with, learn from, and share a decade of my life with. I am truly a very fortunate person because of all that Columbia gave to me."

Hospital, the seventh such program in the country, in collaboration with the College of Physicians and Surgeons. Under his leadership, the program flourished and twenty-five graduates had completed the combined program by 2002.

THE GENERAL PRACTICE RESIDENCY, THE ADVANCED EDUCATION IN GENERAL DENTISTRY, AND PEDIATRIC DENTISTRY PROGRAMS

In addition to the oral and maxillofacial surgery Presbyterian Hospital program, three other hospital dental residencies were initiated or expanded during the 1980s and 1990s. They are the general practice residency (GPR), the advanced education in general dentistry (AEGD), and pediatric dentistry (PD) programs. The growth in the hospital dental programs under Dr. Stephen Roser's leadership during the 1980s and 1990s placed SDOS at the forefront of schools with such programs. These programs enhanced the quality of care for hospital patients and provided opportunity for dental students to gain greater knowledge about how dentists fit into the hospital environment.

Dr. Roser recruited Dr. Ronnie Myers to head up the GPR program, which expanded dental services for special hospital patients who were to receive heart and kidney transplants. The number of GPRs increased to four per year. The general practice residents' hospital-based responsibilities left them little time to treat the patients presenting with more complex dental problems in the main SDOS clinics or to assist in the mentorship of the DDS students who were providing general dental care to patients in the clinics.

To implement the changes in the clinic and undergraduate dental education program envisioned in the strategic plan, it was important to have a cadre of AEGD fellows to interact with faculty practitioners on the one hand and dental students on the other. To accommodate the AEGD program, in the late 1980s, one half of the Vanderbilt Clinic Building (VC) eighth floor was transformed into private practice offices to house the Columbia Dental Associates, the on-site faculty practice program, and the AEGD program. The remaining half of the VC-8 clinic was the third-year DDS clinic. The third-year clinical program for the DDS students was organized around student-faculty groups including AEGD fellows. The AEGD program grew under the leadership of Dr. David Albert and, subsequently, Drs. Stephen Lepowsky, Georgina Zabos, and Greg Bunza. The number of AEGD fellows grew with the assistance of federal grants to twenty-five. Four second-year positions for AEGDs were created to interact with the fourth-year DDS clinic on VC-7. In the mid-1990s a special community-based track was added to the AEGD program to help the school in the development of the Community DentCare program and its network in northern Manhattan (discussed later in this chapter).

Finally, in the 1986–1987 year, with the growth of the hospital dental program, the long-standing university-based postdoctoral training program in pediatric dentistry moved toward a hospital residency when the hospital approved one new residency line in the two-year program in this discipline. By the early 1990s approximately 125 children under age five with extreme oral disease levels were being treated each year in the operating room of Babies and Children's Hospital under the care of the pediatric dentistry faculty and pediatric dentistry residents.

The growth of the hospital dental service provided care, for example, for about fifty cardiac transplant and other organ transplant recipients. In addition, the hospital dental service was able to establish a craniofacial center in the 1990s to bring together the medical and dental disciplines and better coordinate care between a constellation of medical and dental specialists in the surgical treatment and rehabilitation of complex cases of craniofacial deformities and children with cleft lips and palates. None of this would have been possible without the advancement of the oral and maxillofacial surgery program and hospital dental service beginning in the mid-1980s.

THE DENTAL HYGIENE PROGRAM CLOSES

To review, when Columbia University formed the dental school in 1916, the New York School of Dental Hygiene had just been established using facilities of the Vanderbilt Clinic and Hunter College. In 1917 the school was absorbed by Columbia University and renamed "Courses in Dental Hygiene Education." The dental hygiene program continued as a program in the dental school until 1982, establishing a distinguished record over its sixty-three years of existence. The program included a baccalaureate degree program for dental hygienists holding the associate of arts degree, a baccalaureate degree program to train dental hygienists who had completed two years of college or an associate of arts degree, and the first master's degree program in the nation for dental hygienist educators and administrators. For a long period of time the graduates of the latter program became the directors of the majority of dental hygiene programs established in the United States.

Upon Patricia McLean's retirement in 1977, Dona Wayman became the director. Wayman earned her bachelor's and two master's degrees from Columbia; her EdD was also from Columbia. Unfortunately, the

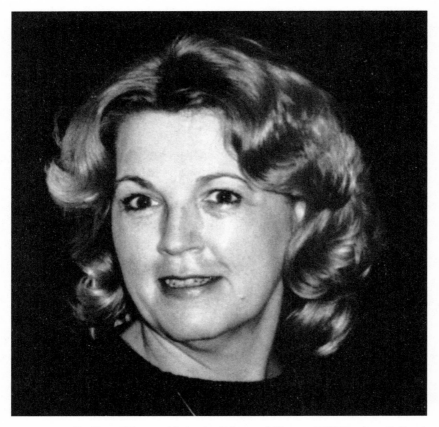

FIGURE 3.5 Dr. Dona Wayman (Columbia BS 1971, MS 1972, EdD Teachers College) served as the director of the Division of Dental Hygiene from 1977 until the program was phased out in 1988.

number of enrolled students at SDOS dropped from more than fifty in 1979 to twenty-six by 1984, and eventually only seven new students enrolled. It was clear why: competition from low-tuition community colleges, which offered dental hygiene training, and the lack of a requirement for the baccalaureate degree for licensure eventually dried up the pool of applicants for Columbia's baccalaureate-level programs who accounted for the majority of enrolled students. The master's-level program was not able to attract a sufficient application pool to sustain dental hygiene education at Columbia. In spite of a valiant effort by Director Wayman and the dental hygiene faculty, the dental hygiene programs were reluctantly phased out in 1987–1988. A similar set of circumstances caused the closure of the dental hygiene programs at other university-based dental hygiene programs in the United States.

THE SCHOOL OF DENTAL AND ORAL SURGERY ENGAGES THE COMMUNITY

The progress made at the school helped to propel it with renewed strength into the twenty-first century. However, there was one more major initiative for the school to undertake under Formicola's deanship: increasing diversity in the profession and improving access to care for minority populations. SDOS's location in northern Manhattan, where communities of color were the majority of the population, provided the school with an opportunity to address some of the problems faced by such communities regarding oral health care. SDOS mapped out a direction to address issues of access to care for the Latino and African American populations in northern Manhattan and to address the lack of diversity in the profession.

SDOS was addressing community issues in the 1990s that would only become apparent to the profession and the public a decade later when the first-ever surgeon general's report on the oral health of the nation was published. The surgeon general, Dr. David Satcher, pointed out in his year 2000 report that while the oral health of the nation was much improved during the twentieth century, the benefits of prevention had not been realized by a large part of the population, such as minority groups and those living in low-income communities. SDOS's early recognition and action regarding the disparity issue established the school's leadership in community health.

During the 1980s and 1990s the school planned and implemented three programs to engage the community and address its oral health problems. They were: the Harlem Hospital-Columbia Postdoctoral Education program, the STEP program, and the Community DentCare program. Together these programs addressed diversity in the profession and access to care. Faculty, students, and staff who participated in these programs enabled the school to address these issues from a community perspective and provided opportunity for a new setting for student learning and faculty research. As a result of these programs, SDOS took a leadership position on the medical campus, in the University, and nationally and helped shape national initiatives by major foundations in the United States.

THE HARLEM HOSPITAL-COLUMBIA POSTDOCTORAL EDUCATION PROGRAM

Harlem Hospital was a major affiliate of Columbia University, and thus a perfect fit for the postdoctoral education program. Dean Formicola and Dr. James McIntosh (DDS, Meharry 1969, and MPH, Columbia 1975), the director of dentistry at Harlem Hospital, recognized that minority communities were more likely to be more comfortably served by minority practitioners. Under McIntosh's leadership, the Harlem Hospital dental service expanded in the mid-1980s from an oral surgical and emergency dental service to one that offered comprehensive dental care. McIntosh recognized that the hospital had difficulty providing specialty services other than oral surgery. In 1988 Formicola and McIntosh established a far-reaching program to augment the dental staff of the Harlem Hospital. The hospital was to have a full range of minority specialists, so that the people of Harlem would have access to all aspects of dental care, including orthodontics for their children. Working with the Harlem Hospital, the postdoctoral training directors, under the leadership of Dr. Thomas Cangialosi at the school and with the assistance of Dr. Edward Healton, the P&S associate dean for Harlem Hospital, SDOS created a special program to enroll Harlem Hospital general practice residents into the school's specialty training programs. By the year 2000 twenty-three African American and Hispanic graduates of the Harlem Hospital Dental Department's general practice residency program completed postdoctoral specialty studies at Columbia.

Fifteen of the graduates from the special Harlem-Columbia program continued to serve as members of the Harlem Hospital staff well into the new century, and twelve held faculty appointments at the dental school. Harlem Hospital has been able to add new specialty services for Harlem residents, providing a total of well over 25,000 patient visits a year.

Graduates of the Harlem Hospital-Columbia postgraduate program helped the school diversify the faculty and assisted the school in its recruitment of underrepresented minorities to the applicant pool. One of the graduates of the program who completed the MPH degree at the Mailman School of Public Health, Dr. Dennis Mitchell, organized the SDOS Office of Diversity and followed up with initiatives begun earlier by Dr. Albert Thompson, an African American alumnus of the class of 1960. Dr. Thompson met with Dean Formicola early in his tenure and explored with him how the school could play a leadership role in making opportunities available for minority students at Columbia. This subject is discussed more thoroughly in Chapter 6.

ALUMNI VOICES: JOHN EVANS

The Harlem Hospital-Columbia University postdoctoral program educated outstanding general practice residents from the Harlem Hospital Dental Service in the postdoctoral specialty programs at Columbia. Dr. John Evans is one of the twenty-three such individuals who were accepted into the program. Dr. Evans now serves as a full-time assistant professor of clinical dental medicine in the Division of Prosthodontics at the College of Dental Medicine. In 2015 he received the Edward V. Zegarelli Teaching Award for excellence in teaching.

Evans was raised in Queens, New York, and commuted to Bernard Baruch College in Manhattan. After earning his BA degree there, he attended the Howard University College of Dentistry in Washington, D.C., where he was awarded the DDS degree in 1983. Evans returned to New York for the residency program in general dentistry at Harlem Hospital. He thinks that Dr. James McIntosh, the director of the Harlem Hospital dental service, recommended him for the specialty program in prosthodontics because "I would study, and work very hard to take advantage of this great opportunity." And Evans really did work very hard. He not only completed the certificate program in the spe-cialty of prosthodontics at SDOS but also completed an additional year at the Bronx Veteran Administration Hospital to learn maxillofacial prosthetics, a highly specialized area of practice that rebuilds orofacial structures lost from cancer or from accidents with intricate prosthetic replacements.

Evans recalls that paying back his loans from dental school and college and living expenses made it difficult for him to attend the special program at CDM. However, "the tuition waiver program and the salary paid by the hospi-tal . . . were wonderful, and greatly appreciated gifts" that made it possible. He credits a long list of "outstanding educators" at the College of Dental Medicine with providing "outstanding instruction," and says that he was "very fortunate to meet and study with students from the other specialty programs." Since entering the special Harlem Hospital-Columbia program in 1992, Evans has grown into an outstanding educator himself, instructing dental and specialty students at CDM. He and other individuals who attended the program have provided much-needed specialty services to the community at Harlem Hos-pital and have become respected and talented members of the CDM faculty.

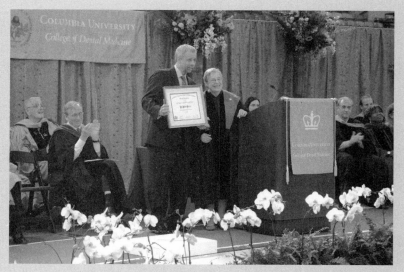

FIGURE 3.6 Dr. John Evans (DDS, Howard 1983) is one of the graduates of the Harlem Hospital-Columbia postdoctoral specialty program in prosthodontics who joined the full-time faculty. He received the Edward Zegarelli Excellence in Teaching Award at the College of Dental Medicine graduation ceremony in 2015.

THE SCIENCE AND TECHNOLOGY ENTRY PROGRAM

Another educational initiative in community engagement was the Science and Technology Entry Program (STEP), a broad community program to help improve high school graduation rates for at-risk students. In 1985 SDOS was the first graduate school in the state to be awarded a New York State STEP grant. The program worked with students from the local communities in grades 7–12 to help improve the high school graduation rate in New York City schools and to encourage students to go on to college with the hope that some would continue on into dentistry. Over the subsequent years, more than 200 students gained academic enrichment each weekend during the school year and during a six-week summer program. The program, under the direction of Dr. Marlene Klyvert, reported that of 102 students who completed STEP from seventh to twelfth grade, 50 percent went on to graduate from college, 8 percent completed a master's degree, and another 4 percent

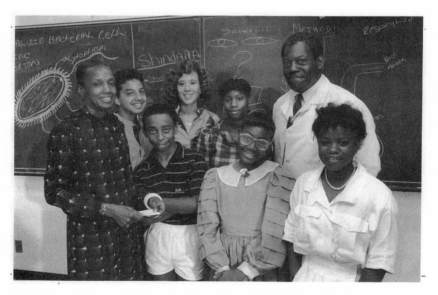

FIGURE 3.7 Science and Technology Entry Program (STEP) students from northern Manhattan at the Columbia University Medical Center with Dr. Albert Thompson, SDOS faculty member (back right), and Margaret Haynes (left front), director of the Office of Minority Affairs at the College of Physicians and Surgeons (ca. 1985).

attended college but did not graduate. While so far it appears that only one of these students will pursue dentistry as a career, the school used its resources and the state grant to help the surrounding communities address a major social issue, improving high school graduation rates and encouraging students to continue on to college.

THE COMMUNITY DENTCARE PROGRAM

The Community DentCare program was planned as a service program for children and senior citizens. It grew out of a 1992 report from the Harlem Prevention Center, a center in the Mailman School of Public Health. The report listed access to dental care as the number one health access issue confronting residents, according to a house-to-house survey of northern Manhattan.

As early as 1986 the school began to increase the services available in the community in conjunction with the development of the Presbyterian Hospital's neighborhood primary-care network, the Ambulatory Care Network (ACN). As a start, Dr. David Albert established a dental practice in the Broadway ACN site. Unfortunately, the hospital did not wish to include dentistry in the other eight primary care sites it established in northern Manhattan over the next fifteen years, even though it was clear that more were needed. So the dental school was basically left to develop a community-based program on its own.

To address this need, in 1996 the school established the Community DentCare program. The aim was to confront the access to care issue identified in the survey and to respond to letters from the principals of public schools sent to Dean Formicola requesting assistance for children with severe toothaches. With the assistance of a $1.2 million start-up grant from the W. K. Kellogg Foundation, SDOS created the Community DentCare Network.

In order to be successful in this endeavor, SDOS hired faculty with additional degrees in public health. As one of the few dental schools in the nation on a health science campus with a school of public health, SDOS committed itself to grow this portion of the faculty. In 1992 the school recruited a senior leader, Donald Sadowsky, DDS, PhD (sociomedical sciences) to rebuild the Division of Community Health. Dr. Sadowsky had many colleagues in the Columbia School of Public Health, as he had earned his degree in public health there. Dr. Sadowsky was able to bring together a core group of faculty to lay the foundation for the school's public health efforts. Later, in 2000, Dr. Burton Edelstein was appointed director of the Division of Community Health and further expanded the division's research and education programs.

Along with the growth of faculty in community health, the school began a strong effort to address the gap in dental services in northern Manhattan. By the year 2001 the DentCare Network consisted of seven public school screening and prevention programs. Two included full treatment facilities, and four included treatment sites in community -based health centers—including one planned and built by the dental school, the Thelma C. Davidson Adair Medical/Dental Center in central Harlem—and a mobile dental van, operated in conjunction with the Children's Aid Society. In total, these programs provided more than 36,000 patient visits to the community in the 2000–2001 year. The leadership and talents of Dr. Stephen Marshall, Dr. Dennis Mitchell, and Dr. David Albert, who worked with multiple partners, made this program a success and a vital resource for the school and the community. While the primary goal of the network was to bring needed services to the residents of Harlem and Washington Heights/Inwood, opportunities to

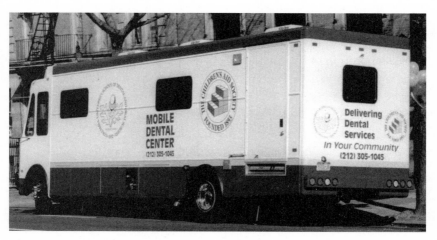

FIGURE 3.8 The first mobile van used by the Community DentCare Network to reach Head Start children. The mobile van program was a collaboration with the Children's Aid Society.

educate postdoctoral general dentistry fellows and elective dental students followed, as the network developed and spawned new research investigations.[7]

The program had several community champions who assisted the school in establishing the Community DentCare program. One special person, Thelma C. Davidson Adair, pointed out that the program in the Harlem community should have some focus on the elderly, as they had had poor access to oral health care for a long time. In addition to the school and van program for children, SDOS created a clinical practice in the heart of Harlem in a historic building, the Mannie L. Wilson Senior Tower. The building was previously the Syndenham Hospital, a hospital that was closed by the Edward Koch administration over the strenuous objections of the community. The dental center geared toward seniors offered medical and dental care and was named for Thelma C. Davidson Adair. Adair was and is a leading citizen in Harlem and became a spokesperson for the good works of this center. Unfortunately, due to financial reasons, it was necessary to transfer the center to the Ryan Center, a federally qualified health center (FQHC). As an FQHC, the Ryan Center had enhanced financial resources for patient care unavailable to Columbia. This made it possible to keep the center afloat.

The Community DentCare program, jointly planned with local community-based organizations and leadership from leading citizens and clergy, became a model for attracting national foundation–funded initiatives to improve health care in underserved communities. With the collaboration of the Mailman School of Public Health, the DentCare program expanded to become the Northern Manhattan Community Voices Collaborative (NMCVC). It attracted a five-year $4.5 million W. K. Kellogg Foundation grant, one of what the foundation called thirteen learning laboratories across the United States and the only one led by dentistry. Later, additional grants totaling more than $3 million continued the program support for five more years. The program brought together thirty-five community-based organizations with faculty from the health sciences schools and leaders in the New York Presbyterian Hospital to improve the health of the community through education and prevention programs. The accomplishments of the NMCVC were documented in a book entitled *Mobilizing the Community for Better Health: What the Rest of America Can Learn From Northern Manhattan.*[8]

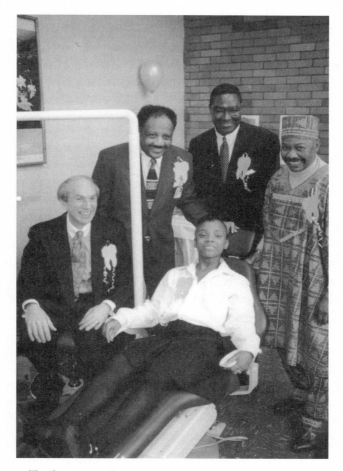

FIGURE 3.9 The Community DentCare Network included several school-based preventive and treatment clinics. Shown here is the opening of a school dental clinic at IS 136 in Harlem with a student trying out the new dental chair (ca. 1996). From left to right: Dean Formicola, Dr. James McIntosh, Dr. Dennis Mitchell, and the head of the Harlem Hospital Community Advisory Board.

In the year 2000 the DentCare program also served as the model for the largest demonstration program ever undertaken in dentistry. Three foundations—the Robert Wood Johnson Foundation, the California Endowment, and the W. K. Kellogg Foundation—teamed up with Columbia. Under the leadership of Dean Formicola and Howard Bailit, a colleague at the University of Connecticut Health Science Center, the team created a program, Pipeline, Profession & Practice: Community-Based Dental Education (Dental Pipeline). The Dental Pipeline program funded twenty-three dental schools in the nation to develop off-site community-based clinical educational experiences in underserved areas for students. These schools were also required to increase their recruitment and enrollment of underrepresented minority students. Columbia served as the national program office, providing the leadership and direction for this combined $27 million initiative of the three foundations.

President George Rupp highlighted the cooperative minority postdoctoral specialty program with Harlem Hospital and the Community DentCare program in his year 2000 report. Upon Formicola's retirement from the deanship, a *New York Times* article reviewed some of the community initiatives begun during his tenure. The article quoted Paul Dunn, the then vice president of Harlem Congregations for Community Improvement. Dunn said, "He's [Formicola] created the template [for community involvement] . . . Hopefully, Columbia will continue the legacy."[9] Upon completing his deanship in 2001, Formicola continued to address the health of the community through a health sciences faculty center he developed called the Center for Community Health Partnerships.

A PRODUCTIVE LONG RUN ENDS AFTER TWENTY-THREE YEARS

During the twenty-three-year period of his deanship, Formicola was able to address the three challenges that he presented in his letter to the vice president of health sciences in 1978: program review, growth of the faculty, and enhancing the financial base of the school. This could not have occurred without the strong support of the faculty and staff at the school; three University presidents, William McGill, Michael Sovern, and George Rupp; the P&S deans and vice president for health science, Paul Marks, Donald Tapley, Henrick Bendixin, Robert Goldberger, Thomas Q. Morris, Robert Levy, and Gerald Fischback; and members of their administration who all assisted the school at various critical points over these years. They became the champions for the school when things were difficult and supported the efforts to continue strengthening the School of Dental and Oral Surgery within the Medical Center

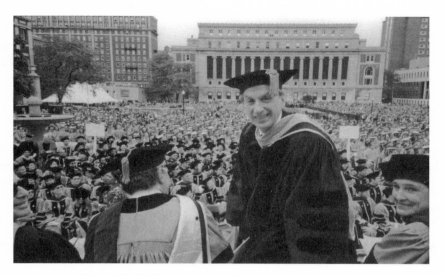

FIGURE 3.10 Dean Allan J. Formicola at the Columbia University Commencement just after presenting his twenty-third and last class of SDOS graduates to the University president for their diplomas in 2001.

and University. The close relationships with the deans of the schools of public health and nursing, Allan Rosenfield and Mary Mundinger, solidified a team approach to problem solving that helped each of these schools advance during this period of time.

In 1991 SDOS paused to mark its seventy-fifth anniversary. The school had much to celebrate, including the successful completion of its $7.5 million capital campaign. A time capsule was locked into a cabinet to be opened on the 100th anniversary of the school in 2016. Two faculty wives, Joyce Goodman and Zel Rubins, with director of alumni affairs Melissa Welsh, created a gala event at the Rotunda in Low Library at which faculty, alumni, and staff took time to celebrate the progress the school had made over its history. Ten years later, a wonderful gala to celebrate Formicola's deanship was also held at the Rotunda in Low Library. It was scheduled for September 29, 2001, just weeks after the awful events of 9/11. Even while the city was still in shock, more than 400 individuals turned out to celebrate the school's accomplishments over the past two decades of the twentieth century.

CHAPTER FOUR

2001–2013: The New Millennium

The School of Dental and Oral Surgery Becomes the College of Dental Medicine[1]

The long and active deanship of Allan Formicola, which lasted twenty-three years, led to a period of growth and stability of the School of Dental and Oral Surgery. Three positive accreditation site visits and reports erased the past problems with the Commission on Dental Accreditation (CODA). Senior faculty, largely drawn from the SDOS World War II–period classes, were replaced with new leadership and a strengthened cadre of junior faculty who were recruited. Many educational changes were put into place, community initiatives were expanded, and advances in patient care programs were undertaken. However, despite a start in strengthening the research mission, much more needed to be done to realize the potential of the school in the research-intense Medical Center and University. In addition, the school needed more expansion space. The competition from other dental schools for the top students had intensified, and the school had to continue forward progress to attract the best students. Formicola recognized that it was time to pass the torch.

In June 2000 Allan Formicola announced he was retiring as dean of the SDOS. He agreed to remain in his position until a successor was identified. There was a prolonged delay in identifying the new SDOS dean, since Dr. Herbert Pardes, the dean of the College of Physicians and Surgeons and the executive vice president for health sciences at Columbia, left his position in 1999 to become president and CEO of the

New York–Presbyterian Hospital. A successor to Dr. Pardes needed to be identified before a new dean of the SDOS could be appointed. In March 2001 the University announced that Dr. Gerald Fischbach, the director of the National Institute of Neurological Disorders and Stroke of the National Institutes of Health, would become the next dean of the College of Physicians and Surgeons and vice president for health affairs. At that moment, the search for the new dean of SDOS could begin in earnest, with Dr. Thomas Morris, who had served as president of the Presbyterian Hospital and interim dean of P&S and vice president, appointed as chair of the search committee.

In September 2001 Dr. Ira Lamster was selected as the next dean, with his appointment commencing in October 2001. Lamster earned his bachelor's degree from Queens College in 1971. He received an SM degree from the University of Chicago in 1972, and the DDS degree in 1977 from the State University of New York, Stony Brook, School of Dental Medicine. He continued on for postdoctoral education in periodontology at the Harvard School of Dental Medicine and earned a certificate in that field and an MMSc degree from Harvard University in 1980. Prior to being recruited to the SDOS, Dr. Lamster was an associate professor of dentistry at the Fairleigh Dickinson College of Dental Medicine. Dr. Lamster began his career at Columbia in 1988, serving as director of the Division of Periodontics, a position he held until 1998. He was then appointed as vice dean of the dental school until he became dean. In addition to conducting a private dental practice in New Jersey, Lamster had accomplished much in the field of dental research (Chapter 3). He had built a robust research program while director of the Division of Periodontics and was well recognized through a strong publication record.[2]

PLANNING WITH THE FUTURE IN MIND

The new dean faced many issues immediately: an upcoming accreditation visit; the academic and administrative structure, finances, and strategic growth; and improving communication were all issues requiring his attention. Having been at the school for thirteen years before becoming dean, Lamster was well aware of future directions necessary to keep the school competitive.

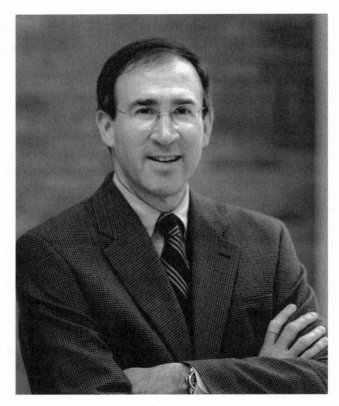

FIGURE 4.1 Dr. Ira Lamster served as dean from 2001 to 2013. Lamster earned his DDS in 1977 from SUNY Stony Brook and a certificate in periodontics and an MMSc from Harvard. He came to Columbia in 1988 as director of the Division of Periodontics and served for three years as vice dean prior to his selection as dean.

Accreditation

The most pressing and immediate issue in late 2001 was the school's accreditation site visit by the CODA, which was scheduled for the following September. The predoctoral program and four postdoctoral programs (endodontics, orthodontics, periodontics, and prosthodontics) were being reviewed. While serving as vice dean, Dr. Lamster had been one of the cochairs of the steering committee preparing the school for accreditation. However, after his appointment as dean, he appointed Drs. Martin Davis and Letty Moss-Salentijn as cochairs for the site visit.

The CODA accreditation site visit went well, with many positive out-comes, and continuation of full accreditation. During Lamster's dean-ship, the school would also make significant advances in carrying out a new strategic plan for the school while facing challenges revolving around financial issues.

Academic and Administrative Structure

The school had prepared a self-study report, as required by the accred-iting agency. This report was used to launch a strategic planning effort for SDOS, which was completed in the first half of 2003. The strategic plan initially focused on changes to the academic and administrative structure of SDOS, with a goal of improving the general organiza-tion of the school and planning for the future. Prior to this reorga-nization, the administrative structure of the school was unwieldy and included ten divisions (roughly equivalent to departments at other dental schools), with four of the ten divisions grouped into two sections, while the other six divisions stood alone. The new table of organization included five sections: (1) adult dentistry (including the Divisions of Operative Dentistry and Prosthodontics); (2) growth and development (the Divisions of Orthodontics and Pediatric Dentistry); (3) hospital dentistry (the Divisions of Oral and Maxillofacial Surgery, and Oral Pathology); (4) oral and diagnostic sciences (the Divisions of Periodontics, Endodontics, and Oral Biology); and (5) social and behavioral sciences (the Division of Community Health, with plans for development of other divisions).

On the administrative side, six associate deans were named for aca-demic affairs, clinical affairs, extramural programs, finance, research affairs, and student and alumni affairs. A number of assistant deans were also identified (special projects and multicultural affairs, post-doctoral programs, extramural hospital programs, and informational resources). Over the eleven years of Dean Lamster's leadership, this structure remained in place, with some additional divisions being cre-ated and some changes in administrative titles reflecting new responsi-bilities. However, while the recommendations from the strategic plan were beginning to steer the school in new directions, the first of the financial challenges had to be faced.

Financial Issues and Fund-Raising

Beginning in mid-2003, the New York State Department of Health announced the intention to change all Medicaid benefits, including dental benefits, to a managed-care format. This would first take effect in the southern part of New York State and would have a dramatic, adverse financial impact on SDOS due to the large percentage of Medicaid patients treated at SDOS (more than 50 percent). This change would mean a shift away from the favorable institutional per-visit rate to a lower capitated rate.

The deans of the five New York State dental schools traveled to Albany on a very regular basis during the last half of 2003 to advocate for an exemption. Assemblyman Richard Gottfried introduced a bill (A5582) that would support the importance of access to dental services and, in essence exempt, or "carve out," the academic dental centers from the transition to Medicaid managed care. The bill passed the Assembly and Senate, and was awaiting Governor George Pataki's signature. The governor, however, had received mixed messages from his advisors regarding the wisdom of enacting the "carve out." Dean Lamster brought the deleterious effect of the change, and the importance of A5582, to the attention of University president Lee Bollinger. He urged Bollinger to contact Pataki's office to request the governor's support. On November 19, 2002, Governor Pataki signed the bill. Columbia's efforts in achieving this end were acknowledged within the New York State Academic Dental Centers group. This is a collaborative effort of the five academic dental centers in New York State (SUNY Buffalo, SUNY Stony Brook, Columbia University, New York University, and Eastman Dental Center). The potential negative impact had this bill not been signed was calculated to be a loss of approximately $2.5 million per year to SDOS for treating the large population of Medicaid patients seen in the clinics. The signing of this bill was a significant achievement for the school and was recognized as such within the Medical Center and University. With this challenge settled, the school could direct its attention to the strategic plan for its future.

The SDOS announced its fund-raising campaign in parallel with the announcement of a Columbia University Medical Center capital campaign. The SDOS campaign was directed toward five goals: renovation of the clinical care areas, providing support to increase the diversity of the SDOS predoctoral class, faculty development, growth of the research mission, and development of a program for oral health care for older adults.

The success of the "carve out" bill led to a continued close working relationship with the New York State legislature and the state government. In March 2004 SDOS received a special legislative grant in the amount of $420,000, which provided support for the dental services program at SDOS. The school would receive additional special allocations from the New York State legislature over the following eight years.

During the first half of 2006, the capital campaign moved into high gear. The fund-raising efforts were invigorated by a gift of $1 million to SDOS from Dr. Samuel Pritz, SDOS/CDM, class of 1933.

The year 2008 also saw new successes in fund-raising. The New York State Assembly gave the SDOS a $1 million grant to expand the Community DentCare program through a renovation of the clinic at the Edward W. Stitt School on 164th Street and a purchase of a new dental van to provide outreach services throughout northern Manhattan and the Bronx. In addition SDOS received a $2.8 million grant from the New York State Health Care Efficiency and Affordability Law (HEAL) program to renovate its patient intake and emergency services areas on the seventh floor of the Vanderbilt Clinic. Another notable gift was received from New York Yankee star ballplayer Alex Rodriguez, who committed $250,000 through his ARod Foundation to support children's oral health and the operation of the SDOS dental van.

The total support provided for capital projects at SDOS between 2008 and 2012 was $14.8 million. By the conclusion of the capital campaign on June 30, 2012, a total of $21 million had been raised, surpassing the original goal by $5 million. This total did not include funds received from New York State or the federal government (research support from the National Institutes of Health). Despite these successes, the school would continue to experience financial stress throughout this era.

Strategic Growth

In 2004 the strategic plan that followed the September 2002 CODA accreditation visit was finalized and disseminated. The plan called for growth of the research mission and significant, strategic growth of the patient care and education missions. In mid-2004 an initiative was announced to develop a program that addressed the three missions, focusing on oral health care for older adults. The growing number of adults sixty-five years of age and older, the trend toward retention of natural teeth for a lifetime, and the absence of any dental benefits in the Medicare program underscored this issue as a major challenge for the dental profession in the next half century. Dean Lamster highlighted this agenda in an editorial published in the May 2004 issue of the *American Journal of Public Health*.[3] An event held at the Columbia University Medical Center on May 4, 2004, focused attention on this issue, and an initiative on geriatric oral health, called ElderSmile (see the "Serving the Underserved: Elders and Kids" boxed text), was announced. This effort, and the editorial published in the *AJPH*, received a great deal of national attention.

SERVING THE UNDERSERVED: ELDERS AND KIDS

An initiative, known as the ElderSmile program, led by Dr. Stephen Marshall, introduced many innovative patient care, research, and education programs associated with the provision of oral health-care services for older adults. The ElderSmile program was soon housed in a state-of-the-art dental site that opened in 2006 at the Isabella Geriatric Center in northern Manhattan. This was a collaborative effort of the SDOS, the Isabella Geriatric Center, and the Henry Schein Company. Following the opening of the clinic, SDOS faculty and trainees provided dental care to the residents. The ElderSmile program also began an outreach effort to seniors attending community senior centers in northern Manhattan. Attendees were offered an oral screening, and those in need of dental care were helped to find locations where affordable care was available. Transportation was provided to those who needed this service. This effort was supported by grants from foundations (the Fan Fox and Leslie R. Samuels Foundation) and corporations.[4]

In 2007 many of the programs previously introduced at SDOS expanded and received local and national attention. The American Dental Association–sponsored Give Kids a Smile Day at the beginning of February, which focuses on provision of services to underserved children, was marked by widespread

SDOS participation. The increased prominence of this national event highlighted SDOS's commitment to the underserved through the DentCare program, which had been introduced nearly twenty years earlier (1988). Further, the focus on geriatric oral health care was highlighted by an information session in Albany sponsored by leaders of the New York State Assembly and Senate. Dr. Lamster and Dr. Cyril Meyerowitz, director of the Eastman Dental Center at the University of Rochester School of Medicine and Dentistry, hosted the event.

In 2008 Dr. Lamster and Dr. Mary Northridge (of the Mailman School of Public Health) published a book titled *Improving Oral Health for the Elderly*.[5] This book, accompanied by the success of the ElderSmile program, firmly established CDM as a leader in oral health care for older adults. The book included contributions from many Columbia faculty members. The recognition of the importance of the growing older adult population was further highlighted by the selection of Dr. Linda Fried as the new dean of the Mailman School of Public Health. Dr. Fried is a geriatrician and an outstanding researcher in geriatrics. The research component of the ElderSmile program expanded with new studies examining the relationship of oral disease to dementia, periodontal disease as a risk factor for ischemic stroke, and the interrelationship of diabetes mellitus and oral health. These studies were supported by the National Institute for Dental and Craniofacial Research, corporations, and foundations and were interdisciplinary projects involving faculty from SDOS, P&S, and the Mailman School of Public Health.

Improving Communications

At about this same time, in 2004, the school launched an initiative to improve communication with the SDOS alumni. Surveys and focus groups revealed that the alumni generally felt they did not have current information about the school, so a two-pronged outreach program was launched. It included improved communication with the annual publication of an alumni magazine (known as *Primus*) complemented by two expanded newsletters (*Primus Notes*) and periodic electronic updates (*ePrimus*). This effort was aimed at better connecting the alumni with the school and seeking their support for the expanding range and breadth of new research, education, and service programs. The second part of this general outreach plan included development of a number of alumni groups and increased visits by the dean and other SDOS faculty to meet with alumni. In the tri-state area, groups were created in New York City, Nassau and Suffolk Counties, Rockland and Westchester Counties, and New Jersey. This outreach effort included regular visits by Dean Lamster to Washington, D.C., Boston, southern Florida, and California to meet with groups of alumni in those regions.

Global Outreach Initiative

In 2005 SDOS began to build a global outreach initiative to promote collaborations with international dental schools. The global outreach was in line with a University initiative in the same direction. The program encompassed scholarly activities, continuing education programs, and plans to provide oral health-care services in selected underserved areas in different countries. As an important benefit, these clinical programs offered SDOS predoctoral students, postdoctoral students, and hospital residents the chance to learn about the delivery of oral health care in other countries and provided trainees with the opportunity to care for persons in different countries who had no access to oral health-care services. As a general measure of the success of the international outreach program, 75 percent of graduating dental students at Columbia had participated in an international experience by 2011.

Japan was one of the first countries in the program. In June of 2005 SDOS signed an education and research partnership agreement with Osaka Dental University in Japan. In keeping with the larger Columbia University global outreach program, this agreement was announced on the Columbia University website's home page.

In that same year, a formal agreement was established with the Faculty of Dentistry at Kuwait University. This program focused on multiyear training of Kuwait University dental graduates who were interested in an academic career in general dentistry. This four-year course of study offered young faculty participation in the Advanced Education in General Dentistry clinical program, and a research program leading to an MS in oral biology. In addition, faculty from SDOS would travel to Kuwait to participate in educational and research activities.

A further affiliation with the Millennium Villages Project, an ambitious program at the Earth Institute of Columbia University to provide

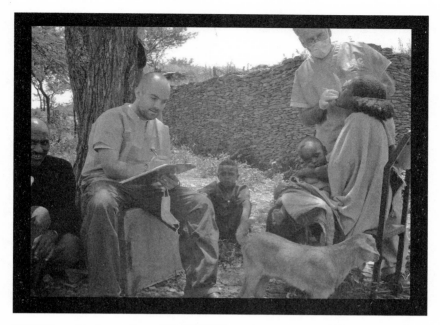

FIGURE 4.2 Dr. Steven Syrop (SDOS, DDS 1980) carrying out a field examination in Ethiopia as part of the global initiative. Jeff Laughlin, a dental student, records the information, while others, including a goat, look on.

broad assistance to countries in sub-Saharan Africa, was also announced. This collaboration led to oral health surveys and provision of emergency care in five countries.

THE SCHOOL OF DENTAL AND ORAL SURGERY BECOMES THE COLLEGE OF DENTAL MEDICINE

Given the changes in dentistry from mainly a surgical field to one that was more preventive and reflective of oral medicine, the School of Dental and Oral Surgery had debated changing its name for some time. In keeping with this shift, by early 2006 SDOS officially changed its name to the College of Dental Medicine (CDM). This change was preceded by a broad communication effort to inform alumni, current students, and the University and Medical Center administration of this intended change and the reasons for the change. In general, the Columbia community was very supportive of the change, which acknowledged the dental school's focus on oral health as a component of overall health. The following message was sent out to the CUMC community after the Columbia University Board of Trustees approved the name change in January 2006.

Dear Columbia University Medical Center Community,

Today, the role of dentists goes far beyond the old perception of someone you visit just when you need a cavity filled. Increasingly, dental research and clinical care has shown that oral health is central to patients' total health. With this focus in mind, the Trustees of Columbia University have approved the renaming of Columbia's dental school to the College of Dental Medicine.

For nearly 90 years, our school, formerly known as the School of Dental and Oral Surgery, has been a national leader in dental education, community service, and research.

Our new name reflects the College of Dental Medicine's comprehensive biomedical approach and its close work with other disciplines in the medical field. Dental faculty and students work side by side with our colleagues from a wide range of disciplines at Columbia University Medical Center and around the world, and are tackling oral health issues from clinical, research and public policy approaches.

A biomedical focus has long been central to our curriculum, as Columbia's dental school students take the same first two years of basic science classes as do P&S students.

Researchers at the College of Dental Medicine are exploring the influence of oral infection on cardiovascular and cerebrovascular diseases, adverse pregnancy outcomes, and diabetes mellitus. From a public health perspective, we are pursuing innovative smoking cessation programs for dental patients and an improved understanding of social determinants of oral health and disease. The College is also leading the effort to address the unique oral health care needs of older adults.

We also run extensive community service health programs in Washington Heights—a federally designated medical and dental manpower shortage area—that afford students rich learning opportunities by exposing them to a broad range of oral health issues. Dental programs in seven area public schools, a dental van that provides oral health screenings and treatment, and three community-based dental clinics, are among the programs marking the College's long heritage of commitment and involvement in the local community.

We hope you will join us in celebrating our new name and continuing collaborative research and clinical environment here at Columbia University Medical Center.

Ira B. Lamster, D.D.S, M.M.Sc.

Following this announcement, for the first time the dental school was identified on the outside of the Presbyterian Hospital building. A pylon with a sign noting the location of the "College of Dental Medicine" was erected next to the circular driveway on 168th Street. This was a small but significant event, since prior to this time there had never been any external signage identifying the dental school at the Medical Center.

A reception was held on April 10, 2006, to officially celebrate the name change. Dr. Fischbach had stepped down in 2005, and at that event, Lee M. Goldman, MD, was introduced as the next dean of the College of Physicians and Surgeons and executive vice president for health and biomedical sciences. Dr. Goldman had previously been the chair of the Department of Medicine at the University of California, San Francisco, School of Medicine.

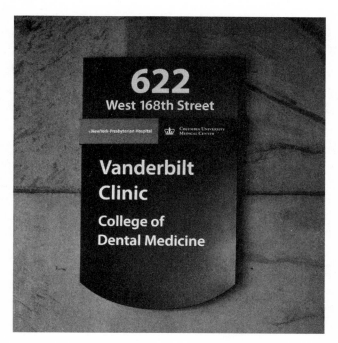

FIGURE 4.3 In 2006, for the first time since the dental school moved to 168th Street in 1928, an outside sign identifies the historical location of the College of Dental Medicine in the Vanderbilt Clinic building.

The changes within the school were not in name only—shifts in leadership, education, and patient care, technological advances, expansions in the faculty and facilities, and more were on the horizon. Dr. Lamster's general outreach to all communities and groups of interest continued, as he was appointed to the New York State Dental Foundation's Board of Trustees. Dr. Lamster was also appointed as chair of the New York State Academic Dental Centers group. In November of 2006 Dr. Lamster was appointed as a senior vice president of Columbia University.

Early 2007 saw an expansion of the continuing dental education program at CDM. Major education programs that were sponsored included oral health care of patients with diabetes mellitus and the relationship of bisphosphonates and osteonecrosis of the jaw (held in conjunction with the New York Academy of Sciences and the Columbia University College of Physicians and Surgeons). The clinical programs, under the leadership of vice dean Ronnie Myers, also were expanding and offering new services. CDM introduced cone beam–computed tomography (CBCT) into the clinic and recruited faculty who were expert in the use of CBCT to lead this new initiative. In midyear, Dr. Lamster's efforts and the commitment of CDM to promote geriatrics and health were recognized by the Isabella Geriatric Center at their annual Raise the Roof Gala.

In the fall of 2007 CDM celebrated its ninetieth anniversary, which was marked by a gala event in October 2007 held at Low Library. This event was accompanied by a display in the main rotunda highlighting the history of the dental profession and dental school at Columbia University. This event was attended by more than 400 people and also acknowledged four distinguished alumni who have contributed greatly to the profession. These individuals included Dr. Irwin D. Mandel (professor emeritus in dentistry), Dr. Susan Karabin (president-elect of the American Academy of Periodontics), Dr. Lawrence Tabak (director of the National Institute of Dental and Craniofacial Research), and Dr. Robert Renner (who developed a nongovernmental organization known as KIDS to provide oral health-care services in the Caribbean and Far East). In addition, eleven members of the faculty and staff with at least twenty-five years of service were recognized.

ALUMNI VOICES: JESSICA LEE

One of the major issues facing dental schools nationally is to encourage graduates to pursue a career in academia. Less than 0.5 percent of the graduates wish to follow in that path, and as a consequence, there is a shortage of qualified, dedicated individuals to fill full-time faculty positions. Jessica Lee (DDS and MPH, SDOS 1997) is one of the exceptions.

She came a long way—from Washington State to New York and Columbia University—after completing college at Western Washington University. Dr. Lee says that she selected the School of Dental and Oral Surgery because of the "joint degree program in dentistry and public health." She notes that the joint degree program is a strength of the school. Talented students using summer and elective times could complete both degrees in four years, and Lee was one such student—she earned both degrees in 1997. She cites Dr. Martin Davis, who was the dean for student affairs and director of pediatric dentistry at the time that Jessica was a student at SDOS, and the then dean (Allan Formicola) as encouraging her to consider a career in academic dentistry.

But her strong Columbia education spurred her on to even greater heights. She accepted a postdoctoral fellowship position at the Cecil G. Sheps Center at the University of North Carolina (UNC) at Chapel Hill, and then in 2002 earned a certificate in pediatric dentistry and a PhD in health policy and management in the Gillings School of Global Public Health at UNC.

Dr. Lee's advancement after accepting a full-time faculty position at the UNC School of Dentistry has been remarkable. She is presently the Demeritt Distinguished Professor of Pediatric Dentistry and the chair of the Department of Pediatric Dentistry at UNC. Jessica has published eighty-six peer-reviewed articles in national journals either as first author or with a team of researchers, a record that most academicians do not achieve in a lifetime of work. The UNC student research group honored her with a Mentor Award and in 2011 the American Academy of Pediatric Dentistry honored her with the Pediatric Dentist of the Year award. In reflecting on her time at Columbia, she said "I loved my time there and thanked the institution for the great academic preparation!" Dr. Jessica Lee exemplifies the type of student Columbia University strives to enroll.

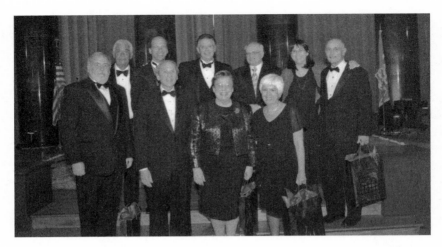

FIGURE 4.4 At the ninetieth anniversary gala in 2007, ten people were honored for their twenty-five years of service to the SDOS, now known as CDM. Front row, left to right: Douglas McAndrew, Allan Formicola, Letty Moss-Salentijn, and Zoila Nougerole. Back row, left to right: Richard Lichtenthal, Ronnie Myers, Martin Davis, David Zegarelli, Stella Efstratiadis, and Thomas Cangialosi.

In 2008 the College opened a new faculty practice site on Haven Avenue. This 2,700-square-foot, state-of-the-art facility replaced the faculty practice in the Medical Center that was in an apartment building on Fort Washington Avenue and did not adequately serve the faculty or their patients. This opening marked an important expansion for the faculty practice that also included two practice locations in the Columbia University Morningside Heights area and a location on East Sixtieth Street between Fifth and Madison Avenues.

In the midst of all these positive changes came a major downturn in the economy, placing many stresses on the CDM budget. The economic stresses, which began in 2008, were felt for the next few years, as the U.S. economy struggled to recover from the Great Recession.

Nevertheless, this time marked a very successful and growth-filled era for the College. A gift from the estate of Harry Levine (SDOS 1936) of more than $1.4 million helped fund the construction of new space assigned to CDM on the seventeenth floor of the Presbyterian Hospital building. This floor housed the Section of Social and Behavioral Sciences, CDM administrative offices, and a large conference room intended for classes, College events, and continuing education courses. In addition, in May of 2009 CDM received the Outstanding Vision—Academic Dental Institution Award from the American Dental Education Association (ADEA) Gies Foundation. This honor was awarded at the 2009 annual ADEA meeting in Phoenix, Arizona.

In September of 2009 CDM had its second full CODA accreditation site visit under Dean Lamster's leadership, and the results were

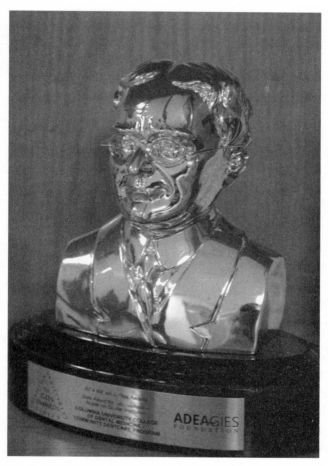

FIGURE 4.5 In 2009 Columbia was awarded the prestigious ADEA award for Outstanding Vision, which was named after William J. Gies, the founder of the Columbia University Dental School and author of the 1926 Carnegie Foundation report on dental education.

outstanding. The predoctoral program and four postdoctoral programs (endodontics, orthodontics, periodontics, and prosthodontics) were reviewed. The predoctoral program received no recommendations, and while "commendations" were no longer awarded, the accreditation steering committee received many positive comments, and the chair of the visiting committee listed seven specific areas of achievement. Three of the four postdoctoral programs received no recommendations, and the fourth received only a single recommendation. The chairs of the CDM steering committee (Letty Moss-Salentijn and James Fine) worked tirelessly to achieve this outcome.

Strengthened Student Body and Curriculum

One of the great strengths of CDM was and is the student body, and the predoctoral students continued to excel in many ways. As an example, Leora Walter, a third-year dental student, received a National Institutes of Health Fogarty International Clinical Research Scholarship-Fellowship. She was the only dental student among the eighty-eight Fogarty-supported trainees. Leora's project examined the prevalence of oral human papilloma virus infection in Peru.

Another important student-related accomplishment at the College during the first decade of the twenty-first century was the dramatic change in the nature of the predoctoral student body, specifically the recruitment of a more diverse class. In 2003 there were a total of twelve underrepresented in dentistry (UID) dental students at the College of Dental Medicine, approximately 4 percent of the student body. By 2012 there were forty-six UID students, representing more than 15 percent of the student body.

This increase in the diversity of the predoctoral class coincided with the entering classes being at the very top of the academic ranking of all dental schools in the United States and was achieved by the appointment of a senior associate dean for diversity and multicultural affairs and the provision of scholarship support for students designated as UID. Dr. Dennis Mitchell, already a full-time faculty member at CDM, became the senior associate dean following reorganization of the College. Dr. Mitchell created a supportive environment that highlighted the importance of diversity, student involvement, and program development at CDM. The Office of Diversity and Multicultural Affairs sponsored programs and provided student support. Further, the CDM administration provided needed scholarship funds to attract students, though the scholarships provided were never as large as ones offered by other dental schools to very outstanding students of color. CDM continued to attract students because of what it offered in terms of the personal and academic environments and exciting opportunities available after graduation.

The class of 2013, which entered CDM in the fall of 2009, was also the first to participate in a new predoctoral curriculum. The new curriculum was conceived in cooperation with the P&S and was true to the College's fundamental commitment to the founding document. It emphasized a strong foundation in biomedical sciences even while shortening the basic sciences schedule to a year and a half and a concentration of preclinical training moved forward into the second semester of the second year. This preclinical training was based on an innovative case concept, with students learning to treat simulated patients with specific problems and not just practicing clinical procedures on typodonts. The new curriculum also included early entry into the clinic, off-site clerkships in general dentistry at affiliated hospitals, and greater translation of the basic sciences into the clinical experiences. This new curriculum was introduced for the class of 2013; the challenge during this period was that the 2010, 2011, and 2012 classes were to complete their education in the "old curriculum," so the college was simultaneously offering two different educational programs for three years.

A NEW RESEARCH COMPLEX

That same year construction began on a major new research complex on the twelfth floor of the Vanderbilt Clinic building. This lab complex, which was constructed in collaboration with the Department of Biomedical Engineering from the School of Engineering and Applied Sciences, was focused on stem cell research. At CDM, Dr. Jeremy Mao, who served as codirector of the Center for Craniofacial Regeneration, led this program. The center's work was truly interprofessional, involving orthopedists, plastic surgeons, biomedical engineers, and dentists, including oral surgeons, orthodontists, and endodontists. Among the

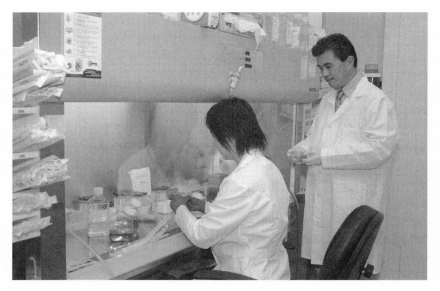

FIGURE 4.6 Dr. Jeremy Mao working in the Tissue Engineering and Regenerative Medicine Laboratory with Dr. Wenli Zhao.

center's oral disease projects were stem cell–based regeneration of the temporomandibular joint and regeneration of dental pulp tissue. This research attracted more than $10 million in funding from the National Institutes of Health, as well as significant corporate support.[6]

Evolution and Advancement

As the end of the first decade of the twenty-first century approached, CDM continued to expand and evolve. Activities associated with the American Dental Association's annual Give Kids a Smile Day (February 5) were centered in New York City and the pediatric dentistry clinic at CDM. Further, CDM's dental implant program was dramatically enhanced with the recruitment of Dr. Dennis Tarnow, a national and international leader in the field, as director of implant education at the College. His appointment was announced on May 1, 2010, and resulted in a dramatic expansion of the clinical training programs at CDM, new research in clinical implantology, and continuing education opportunities for practicing dentists. Dr. Tarnow recruited a large group of volunteer faculty who helped to strengthen both clinical and didactic implant education at the College.

The year 2010 also marked other critically important advances for the College. For the second year in a row, the entering class (of 2014) was the most academically competitive of any dental school class in the United States. The new patient intake area on the seventh floor of the Vanderbilt Clinic, funded by the HEAL grant, was completed. It included a new triage/radiology complex and a separate emergency clinic to treat the thousands of patients with dental emergencies who are seen each year at CDM. The new Center for Dental and Craniofacial Regeneration became operational on the twelfth floor of the Vanderbilt Clinic building and attracted major research support from the NIH. Further, new research programs examining the genetics of periodontal disease and oral squamous cell cancer, were begun. Dr. Panos Papapanou led the periodontal project, and Drs. Angela Yoon and Athanasios Zavras were studying the genetic epidemiology of oral squamous cell cancer. In addition, through the efforts of Dr. Burton Edelstein, the College received

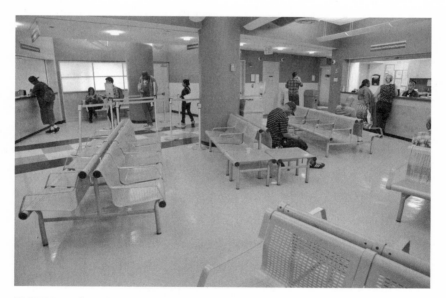

FIGURE 4.7 In 2010 a reconstructed triage/radiology area was opened on the seventh floor of the Vanderbilt Clinic. This is the intake area for thousands of new patients, emergency patients, and patients of record.

major grants from the Health Resources and Services Administration to support public health training for residents in pediatric dentistry and dental students who sought clinical training combined with a public health education (dual-degree DDS–MPH program).

This new funding dramatically increased predoctoral student interest in the DDS–MPH program, and complemented another dual-degree program established during Dr. Lamster's term as dean. Working with Dr. Letty Moss-Salentijn and Dr. Marlene Klyvert, a dual DDS–MA program with Teachers College of Columbia University was developed.

ALUMNI VOICES: JUNE HAREWOOD

The College of Dental Medicine attracts many students from all over the world, including Canada. June Harewood (DDS, 2011, and PD Orthodontics, 2014) is one of the Canadian students. She was raised in Ottawa and received her undergraduate education at the University of Toronto. June selected CDM to study dentistry because of the international opportunities under the college's global initiatives program, the dual-degree program, and the college's excellent reputation. Harewood graduated in 2011 and continued on to complete her postdoctoral education in orthodontics in 2014.

Harewood says that the strengths of her Columbia education were the "opportunities for international global health externships—I went to the Philippines and Ethiopia—the strong focus on treating the patient as a whole, and the excellent basic science/medical education to supplement my dental education." Of Dr. Dennis Mitchell, who was her mentor, Harewood says, "[He] was my guardian angel in every way possible. He encouraged me to pursue summer research projects and facilitated my inclusion in one of his studies. I would never have survived dental school without him!"

In reflecting on her time at Columbia, Harewood says, "Columbia has provided me with an excellent understanding of the dental and medical problems faced by each patient. My education provided me with several opportunities to work in the local Washington Heights/Harlem community, which showed me that I always want to serve underserved populations during my career. I have gained confidence in my own abilities because the faculty at Columbia had confidence in me." Dr. Harewood just completed an orthognathic fellowship at Jacobi Hospital and has accepted a full-time position on the College of Dental Medicine faculty in the Division of Orthodontics.

This program was intended for students with an interest in dental education and was well subscribed. The first dental student to participate in the program was Roseanna Graham who, after graduation from both CDM and Teachers College and completion of a general practice residency, returned to CDM as a member of the faculty. She went on to earn her PhD in science education from Teachers College.[7]

ONGOING FINANCIAL STRESS

Nevertheless, at the close of the first decade of the twenty-first century, the financial stress on CDM remained a critical factor in determining the ability of the College to evolve and develop new programs. Between fiscal year 2001 (FY 2001) and FY 2012, the CDM annual budget increased from $35 million to $56 million. During that period a new formula was developed by the CUMC administration (referred to as the FAIR model), which increased the overhead to the CDM from $4.9 million in FY 2001 to $11.3 million in FY 2011. Hence, the percentage of the CDM budget devoted to overhead increased from 14 percent to more than 20 percent. A survey of other dental schools affiliated with private universities in the Northeast taken at the time that the FAIR model was introduced revealed that CDM's common cost was the highest of all schools. This financial situation made program advancement and new development very challenging.

External changes further influenced the CDM budget. In 2009, with the election of Andrew Cuomo as governor of New York, there was a major overhaul of the state Medicaid system, including the reimbursement program. Prior to this overhaul, reimbursement was based on an institutional rate, which, as noted previously, was carved out of earlier changes to the Medicaid reimbursement program. Under the new administration, the changes included introduction of the ambulatory patient groups method of reimbursement. This rate reform was directed to outpatient services and diagnostic and treatment centers (which is how the dental school clinics were classified). Reimbursement rates were now based on the relative degree of difficulty of the procedures and bundling of services. In the description of the change, the financial effect on providers was intended to be neutral at worst, with an anticipated increase in reimbursement as the Medicaid program intended to shift patient care away from hospitals and into the community. Nevertheless, in an environment in flux, this was another potential stressor, as reimbursement rates needed to be negotiated with managed-care companies, as did direct reimbursement from the state. The program was introduced in 2009, with a phase-in over the first four years.

At this time, CDM was also in the process of changing to an electronic patient record (EPR). The College chose the most commonly used system for dental schools (axiUm). The implementation of the EPR was lengthy and included consideration of different record systems following a call for proposals in 2009, a faculty-wide retreat in 2010, initial rollout in the pediatric dentistry clinic in April 2011, and then full implementation in June 2011. The decision was made to implement both record-keeping and other modules, including the billing component, in the axiUm system in June 2011. Therefore, communication was needed between the College's EPR and the new ambulatory patient groups reimbursement system for Medicaid services. As expected, problems were encountered in the first months, which resulted in a reduction in clinic income in the beginning of the EPR era. This downturn was reversed the following year.

THE BORDER BETWEEN DENTISTRY AND MEDICINE

Columbia's dental school had a long history of championing dentistry's role in relation to medicine in the care of the public, and this question once again came to the fore when Larry Tabak (DDS, SDOS 1977, and PhD, SUNY Buffalo presented this question at a symposium in 2007:

> Will dentists be educated to the highest level, like ophthalmologists, or at a more technical level, like optometrists or will they be concerned only with "looks" as are opticians? . . . Will they fully comprehend the biology of oral health and disease and be capable of treating the most complex conditions? If dental schools are to educate dentists to be the highest-level provider . . . then the schools must build their base of scientific knowledge as well as inspire dedication to scientific research and knowledge among dental students.[8]

At the time of the symposium, Lawrence Tabak was the director of the National Institute of Dental and Craniofacial Research. He currently is the principal deputy director of the National Institutes of Health.

The larger question of how the future of dental education and practice fit into the primary-care system in the United States continued as important themes for CDM and Dean Lamster. Throughout 2011 Lamster made important presentations on this topic to the American Dental Association's Board of Trustees, the annual meeting of the American Dental Education Association, the New York Academy of Sciences, and the annual session of the American Dental Association regarding dentistry's role in primary care. That same year this subject was featured on CBS News and was the focus of a Dunning symposium in New York City.

In addition, Irwin Mandel's legacy at the Columbia University College of Dental Medicine was his research at the border of dentistry and medicine. These contributions were honored at a special memorial service at CDM in September 2011. Speakers included Lawrence Tabak, Dr. Bruce Baum from the National Institute of Dental and Craniofacial Research, Dr. Dan Malamud from the New York University College of Dentistry, and members of the Mandel family.

LAMSTER'S LEGACY

In the spring of 2012 and after eleven years of his deanship, Dean Lamster announced his intention to step down from his position on June 30, 2012. Under his leadership the dental school at Columbia University had successfully managed financial challenges while instituting far-reaching changes during the first decade of the twenty-first century. There were fiscal growth, changes to the physical plant, a new predoctoral curriculum, expansion of the community outreach programs and faculty practice network, and broadening of the research mission. The international outreach program was robust and had become an essential part of the College's activities. The student body was academically gifted and diverse. Alumni relations were at an all-time high, with ever-increasing numbers of alumni attending events and contributing to the College.

Nevertheless, the College still faced significant challenges. The cost of dental education continued to rise, and student indebtedness at graduation was a major determinant of career choice for many students. Outstanding students who might have chosen less lucrative but important careers in education, research, and public health were forced to make choices based primarily on future earnings potential, thus choosing careers in the clinical dental specialties. While the College gained expansion space, it continued to be extremely constricted, with far less space than its peer schools, and needed to renovate one of its core teaching facilities, the preclinical laboratory. Further, the College was faced with a very challenging budget model, encumbered by heavy overhead charges from the Medical Center and University and the very high cost of construction in old buildings with antiquated infrastructure. However, the strength of CDM over its long history has always been its people, and these individuals will continue to work together as the College prepares to celebrate its 100th anniversary.

RONNIE MYERS, THE INTERIM DEAN SETS THE STAGE

After the announcement of Dr. Lamster stepping down as dean there was concern about who Dr. Lee Goldman, the executive vice president for health sciences and the dean of the Faculty of Medicine, would appoint as interim dean. Dr. Goldman sought out the support and leadership of the College of Dental Medicine in deciding whom to appoint as interim dean. In June of 2012, Dr. Goldman announced that Dr. Ronnie Myers would serve as the interim dean while the search for the next dean was conducted. The goal for the interim dean was to set the stage for the next leader of CDM while at the same time creating and maintaining an atmosphere and environment in the CDM for the current students, faculty, and staff to continue their academic endeavors and building upon opportunities, needed growth, and support. Dr. Goldman appointed a search committee to locate the new dean. The search committee was chaired by Dr. Steven Shea, MD, MS, senior vice dean of the College of Physicians and Surgeons, and the search went forward while Dr. Myers served as interim dean.

Dr. Myers, a 1979 alumnus of the SDOS DDS program, earned his certificate in pediatric dentistry from the Columbia program in 1980. He began his full-time role on the faculty in 1982 and thirty years later, on July 1, 2012, he began as interim dean. In previous positions at the

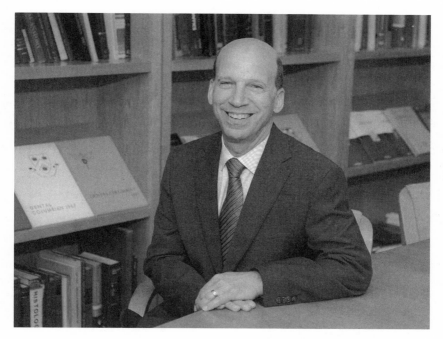

FIGURE 4.8 Ronnie Myers (DDS, SDOS 1979, Pediatric Dentistry, SDOS 1980) was appointed interim dean in 2012 and served until Dean Christian Stohler was appointed in July of 2013. Myers continues to serve as vice dean for administrative affairs.

SDOS/CDM, he served as the clinical dean and the vice dean for administrative affairs. Myers continued in these roles, maintaining his private practice, teaching commitments, and research in infection prevention and HIV testing in the primary oral health-care setting while serving as interim dean.

To pave the way for a new dean, Dr. Myers began several initiatives during his interim deanship. They included: establishing a "True Cost" modeling project in coordination with CUMC so that decentralization of the CDM budget could be developed; hiring a consultant to review the entire clinical organization as a cost center to become more cost accountable and to improve the organizational support for the clinical programs; and beginning discussions to explore the possibility of developing significant off-site clinical programs with two well-established CUMC partners, the Bassett Health System in rural upstate New York and La Clinica de Familia in La Romana, Dominican Republic. Both areas needed oral health services, and the latter is directly related to CDM's patient population, which includes many residents from the Dominican Republic. In addition, the initiatives included establishing a communications group to improve the CDM's website and to enhance the dissemination of information about the local, national, and international work undertaken by students, faculty, and the college. Fund-raising and development activities continued. Initial discussions were held on how the CDM would celebrate its centennial year in 2016–2017. The interim dean had a crowded agenda.

Dean Goldman, the dean of P&S and chief executive of CUMC, also committed to making a site on the CUMC campus available for a new building for CDM during the year. As pointed out in earlier chapters in this history, throughout its 100 years the SDOS/CDM has searched for the best way to expand its facilities. The potential for the construction of a new building was linked with the CDM's financial development. A review and reevaluation of all CDM endowments was carried out so that the new dean would understand the financial potential available for moving CDM forward.

The interim year brought several previous projects to a successful end. The new faculty practice location in the Columbia Doctors location at 51 West Fifty-First Street in midtown Manhattan opened. This new site was larger than the previous site at 16 East Sixty-First Street. The dental practitioners joined practitioners from CUMC primary-care and specialty physician groups. The new Implantology Center on the ninth floor of the Vanderbilt Clinic opened. It is the site for an implant fellowship program and brings all implant surgery together in one location. The newly refurbished Bard athletic facility opened. This refurbishment was the combined effort of all four schools on the CUMC campus: medicine, dentistry, nursing, and public health.

In September of 2011, as noted earlier, Irwin Mandel's legacy at the Columbia University College of Dental Medicine was honored at a special memorial service at CDM. In April of 2013 on Birnberg Research Day, which celebrates the research accomplishments of our students with a visiting professor, the large conference room on the newly renovated Presbyterian Hospital floor 17-West was named in Irwin Mandel's honor. Mandel had a long and distinguished research career and was the first recipient of the American Dental Association's Gold Medal for Research.

Making sure that there is sufficient assistance to operate the academic and clinical missions of the school is critical to meeting those missions. The administrative and support staff of the College of Dental Medicine provides day-to-day assistance for the administration, faculty, and students. They serve in a variety of capacities, assisting in the dean's office, the academic sections' offices, the alumni, student, and financial affairs offices, and in the offices of the off-site programs. Operating a large and complex clinic program requires dedicated staff. The skills required of staff have become more specialized in the twenty-first century. Zoila Nougerole, the administrative manager in the dean's office, has the important responsibility of hiring and training staff and creating a positive environment for staff to function at a high level. There are now approximately 200 administrative and staff members at the CDM.

Faculty transitions continued during the year, from recruitment to retirement. A search for a microbiologist was successfully completed. Dr. Yiping Han joined the faculty as a tenured professor in the Section of Oral and Diagnostic sciences. Dr. Mildred Embree, DMD, PhD, a full-time tenured faculty member in the Section of Growth and Development, collaborated with other faculty at CUMC to expand her research efforts. Dr. Laureen Zubiaurre Bitzer was promoted from assistant dean of admissions to associate dean for student affairs. Prior to serving in her current role, she served as the director of the third-year DDS clinical program.

Three longtime dedicated faculty members—Drs. Thomas Cangialosi, David Zegarelli, and Martin J. Davis—announced their retirement from Columbia during the year. Dr. Tom Cangialosi (Georgetown DDS, 1959 and SDOS Orthodontics, 1975) the Leuman Waugh Professor of Orthodontics, was the section chair of growth and development and the director of the Division of Orthodontics. He also served the SDOS as the associate dean for student and alumni affairs and as associate dean for postdoctoral education. He was a full-time faculty member for more than twenty-five years and was a past president of the American Board of Orthodontics. Dr. David Zegarelli (1969), at the time of his retirement, was the director of the Division of Oral Pathology. The oral pathology division under David Zegarelli's leadership grew to three full-time faculty members and established a New York Presbyterian Hospital oral and maxillofacial pathology residency program with an optional

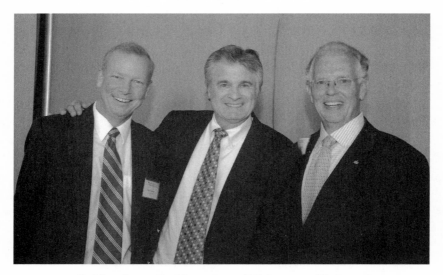

FIGURE 4.9 In May of 2013, Dr. Martin Davis (DDS, 1974 and Pediatric Dentistry, 1975), senior associate dean for student and alumni affairs, retired (right). Here he is seen with his brother far left, Dr. Daniel Zedeker (DDS, SDOS 1983), and longtime friend, fellow alumnus, and colleague Dr. Stuart Epstein (now deceased).

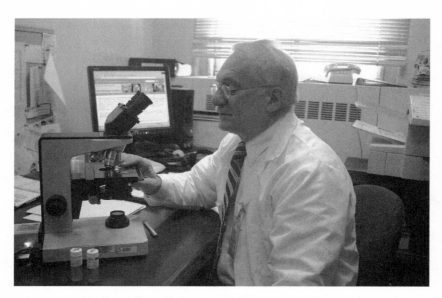

FIGURE 4.10 Dr. David Zegarelli, longtime faculty member and oral pathologist/ medicine, retired in 2013 and was recognized at an alumni reception. Shown here at his microscope, Zegarelli's expertise was widely recognized.

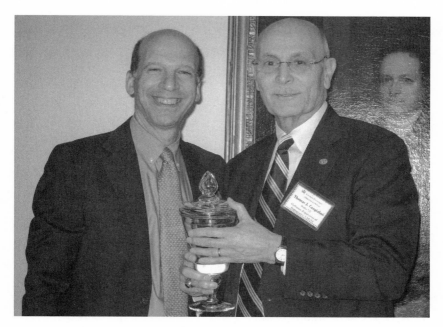

FIGURE 4.11 Interim dean Myers (left) presents a gift to Dr. Thomas Cangialosi on his retirement. Cangialosi served as assistant dean for student affairs in the 1980s and then as director of the Division of Orthodontics and Associate Dean for Postdoctoral Education until he retired.

MD component. Dr. Martin J. Davis (DDS, SDOS 1974 and Pediatric Dentistry, 1975), joined the full-time faculty upon graduation. He served as the director of the Division of Pediatric Dentistry and the senior associate dean of student and alumni affairs. He had a distinguished career that included becoming the president of the American Academy of Pediatric Dentistry and the American Society of Dentistry for Children. During Dr. Davis's long tenure at CDM as senior associate dean of students, he established excellent relationships with students and alumni. Each of these faculty who retired was recognized by CDM during the interim year.

The College had four program site visits by the CODA during Dr. Myers's interim deanship. They included the programs in pediatric dentistry, general practice residency, advanced education in general dentistry, and the initial visit for the newly created residency program in dental public health. All were successfully concluded. The year had some unexpected events. In October, the University endured Hurricane Sandy, during which the University was unprecedentedly closed for two days. In April the CDM dean's office and adjacent offices suffered a flood from a broken ceiling fire sprinkler head that displaced the entire dean's suite for six months until October 2013.

At graduation in 2013, Dr. Myers established a new tradition at the CDM commencement exercises. The graduates recited an "Oath for the Oral Health Professions." Written by Dr. Myers and modeled after the Hippocratic Oath, it acknowledges the special role that graduates of the College of Dental Medicine have in integrating oral health care with primary care and interprofessional collaboration for the well-being of their patients. The new dean would recognize Dr. Myers's dedication and accomplishments as interim dean by continuing him in the role of vice dean for administrative affairs.

The announcement of the new dean, Dr. Christian Stohler, came in June of 2013 with a welcome reception on the twentieth of the month. Thus, the next chapter for the College of Dental Medicine began.

CHAPTER FIVE

2013–2016 and Beyond: Plans for the Next 100 Years

The preceding chapters cover the history of the College of Dental Medicine up until the present time. This chapter aims to record the College's activities during the 2014–2015 academic year and set the stage for the College's plans for the future. Of course, the latter is often said to be difficult to do and a version of the famous quote attributed to Niels Bohr and appropriate to academic institutions is "it is difficult to predict, especially the future" [but] "it might be useful (and fun) to pick out some recent developments which might be the forerunner of things to come."[1] So this chapter will complete the history of CDM and leave to the next generation the predictions or vision that the current generation believes will continually strengthen CDM to meet its original mission as a "dental school on university lines."

A CHANGE IN LEADERSHIP: CHRISTIAN STOHLER SELECTED AS DEAN

If the history of the school has one thing to teach us, it is that changes in the leadership of the institution have led to new initiatives. In this, recent history is no different. During the year that Dr. Ronnie Myers served as interim dean, a search committee to locate a new dean was appointed by Dr. Lee Goldman, the dean of the Faculties of Health Sciences and Medicine and the executive vice president for health and

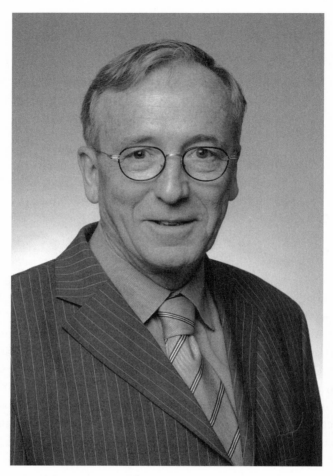

FIGURE 5.1 Christian Stohler was appointed dean of the College of Dental Medicine in 2013. He served as dean of the University of Maryland School of Dentistry for ten years before arriving at Columbia.

biomedical sciences. In August of 2013, Dr. Christian Stohler joined the CDM as the next dean. Stohler was well qualified: he had just served ten years as dean of the University of Maryland School of Dentistry. Prior to this, he spent more than twenty years at the University of Michigan as professor and chair of the Department of Biologic and Materials Science. Christian Stohler received his DMD from the University of Bern in Switzerland where he also earned a DrMedDent in hematology and certificates in oral surgery and prosthodontics. He is an expert on pain management and temporomandibular joint diseases.

Stohler spent the first year of his deanship (2013–2014) carefully reviewing the school and reordering the manner in which the school's budget was managed. He brought the faculty together in several retreats to discuss the school's major programs and possible areas for new directions. He laid the foundation to create budgeting centers at the level of the school's five sections. Budgeting at the section level would make better use of resources and stimulate growth.

THE INTERNAL REVIEW

On October 1, 2014, thirteen months after his appointment, Dean Stohler brought the faculty and student body together in Alumni Auditorium to discuss the state of the school. He reported his findings and pointed to future directions in areas ranging from research

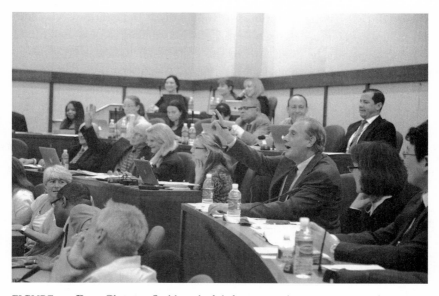

FIGURE 5.2 Dean Christian Stohler scheduled strategic planning retreats to discuss future directions for the College of Dental Medicine. Here the faculty is shown at the School of Social Work on the Morningside campus at one of several retreats. Dr. James Fine (far right in photo) raises a question!

to funding to the composition of the student body to the role of emerging technology.

During his internal review of CDM, Dean Stohler stressed the importance of aligning the College's missions and resources with those of the University and Medical Center. He chose to focus attention on the school's missions in relationship to the culture and ethos of Columbia University. He noted that Columbia University was ranked eighth among the twenty top academically ranked universities in the world. Of those top universities, five have dental schools—Columbia, Harvard, University of California, San Francisco, University of Pennsylvania, and the University of Washington. These are all research-intensive universities. Over the four-year period of 2009–2013, Columbia University was fourth among these universities in receiving funds from the National Institutes of Health. Of the five dental schools, the College of Dental Medicine in the same period was fifth in receiving funds from the NIH.

Another key measure of scholarship is the total number of faculty publications and citations in the literature. In the same period, of the five peer dental schools, Columbia was fifth and close to the publication record of UCSF both in numbers of publications and citations. The dental schools at Harvard and Columbia are the smallest of the five schools. Given the relatively small size of the Columbia University College of Dental Medicine compared with its larger peers, the review indicated that the CDM was going in the right direction regarding its research mission. Stohler's review also noted that in the 2013–2014 year, CDM attracted additional support from commercial companies and foundations to support research and scholarly work. This added $2.5 million to the $9.8 million of NIH support earned in the indexed years.

In his presentation, the new dean highlighted a few of the ongoing research programs funded by the NIH. Dr. Jeremy Mao's research group currently works in the areas of stem cell biology, tissue engineering, and wound healing. Dr. Daniel Oh's research interests are in the areas of biofunctional materials for implantology, regenerative restorative medicine by means of tissue engineering, and nanotechnology. And Dr. Panos Papapanou and colleagues have recently shown that periodontal disease can be classified by genetic markers.

The new dean, having come to CDM with a research background and experience in leading another dental school, was well aware that it takes a continual effort to maintain and expand what he terms high-impact science and research support from the NIH, given the competition for that funding. He recognized that there is room for growth in the research program and that the College should continue to strive for a higher place within its peer group.

In his review Stohler also noted that the College should capitalize on the initiatives of the previous two deans. The College's research emphasis on comorbidity of oral disease and systemic disease under Dean Ira Lamster has led to a reappraisal of the dentist's role in primary care. This aligns with the school's educational emphasis upon joint basic science education for both medical and dental students. Under Dean Allan Formicola, the College also placed emphasis on the social justice mission with the establishment of the Community DentCare Network. This aligns the college with the missions of the hospital and the Mailman School of Public Health. The dean has called for a review of the DentCare program to realign it with the school's educational and research missions and to solidify the academic aspects of the program in the renamed Section on Population Oral Health.

As noted in the student and alumni section of this history in Chapter 6, the dean reported that the college's fund-raising efforts realized $5.1 million in support in the 2013–2014 year. And that, on what is called a Giving Day, it was in second place of the seventeen Columbia schools in the participation of its alumni in that effort! The chair of the 1852 Society, Dr. Thomas Magnani, has pledged assistance in raising new funds to further the efforts of the dean and the College.

Stohler conducted a further external review of the school regarding its competitiveness with respect to peer institutions in the Northeast on the basis of DDS tuition and fees. Stohler found that CDM fares favorably on the four-year costs in comparison with Harvard, UCSF, University of North Carolina, and University of Washington. Costs at CDM were substantially less than that of the four-year costs at New York University (NYU), University of Southern California, the University of the Pacific, and the University of Pennsylvania. Columbia costs are 18 percent lower than the highest-cost school, NYU, and only 10 percent higher that the lowest-cost school, at University of California, Los Angeles. Similarly, the costs for the postgraduate programs in comparison with peer programs are either the first or second lowest.

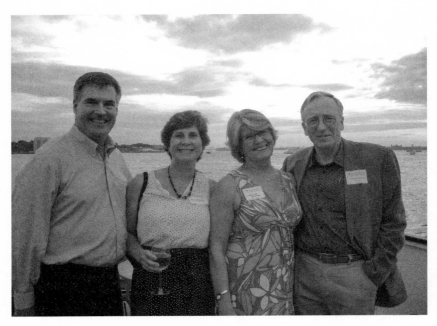

FIGURE 5.3 Dean and Mrs. Christian Stohler (right) with Dr. and Mrs. Thomas Magnani enjoy a Hudson River cruise alumni event. Tom Magnani (DDS, SDOS 1980) has served as chair of the 1852 Society and will head up the centennial campaign.

The class of 2018 of eighty students admitted in the fall of 2014 was selected from 2,056 applicants with high Dental Aptitude Test scores of 23 (the highest score possible in 2013 was 25) and grade point averages of 3.63. As reported in Chapter 6, forty-three students are male, thirty-seven are female, and 20 percent are minority students. The students came from sixteen states and attended fifty-eight different colleges, and there were four international students. Success in acceptance into prestigious postgraduate and residency programs is noteworthy. Greater than 90 percent of graduates in the class of 2014 were accepted into these programs, placing CDM at the top of all schools in this measure.

During the 2014–2015 year there were eighty-two postdoctoral students and twenty-six New York–Presbyterian Hospital residents enrolled in ten programs. There were 102,000 patient visits provided in the dental clinics in the Vanderbilt Clinic building and 12,000 visits provided to children in the dental clinic in the Mailman School of

Public Health building. The Community DentCare program provided an additional 14,000 patient visits to children in public schools and its mobile van.

The internal review of the College in relation to its mission and with a comparison with peers allowed the new dean to decide where to place his emphasis. In moving forward, the dean recognized the stresses placed on the school's resources to move to the next level. The "Columbia brand" of a close interface with the College of Physicians and Surgeons and opportunities for curriculum innovation are hallmarks of the school. Dean Stohler identified several areas of potential strengths that the curriculum could build upon. They are: information age; oral health/dentistry; personalized education and dual degrees; population oral health: rural, urban, and global; comorbid conditions; and interprofessional education. The formation of a "digital dentistry" committee will provide some of the underpinnings for future curriculum innovations and to assist in these efforts.

In envisioning the future of the CDM, Dean Stohler noted that students already arrived at the CDM with a keen understanding of the impact of technology on their futures. The CDM can take a leap forward by incorporating computer hardware in tandem with the application of necessary software to move from the industrial age of dentistry to the information age of dentistry. This will have an impact on every aspect of the school and students' education from the manner in which the curriculum and courses are offered to the technology used in the clinics to deliver patient care. The dean's presentation was optimistic about the future of the College but recognized the challenges to continual success.

So what were the current programs and activities that the new dean found at CDM on which he could build the future? What follows are those programs and activities of the five sections responsible for the educational and patient care programs as described by their leaders during the academic year 2014–2015, two years before the 100th year anniversary. Their plans for the future are included. The overall curriculum for the DDS students underwent a major revision just prior to this time and that too is described. In addition, those administering these programs describe the current school initiatives on diversity and inclusion and on outreach service to the community.

THE COLLEGE OF DENTAL MEDICINE CURRICULUM
AND THE SECTIONS' PROGRAMS IN THE 2014–2015 YEAR

The curriculum[2] for the DDS program has been shaped over the past almost 100 years as described in Chapters 1 through 4. The present curriculum (2014–2015) reflects ongoing evolutionary changes. Of note is the shift in the clinical curriculum to a more patient-centered model in which students deliver care to a panel of patients (Chapter 3). The biomedical sciences curriculum recently has undergone major changes. Separate courses in the basic sciences have been integrated, with an emphasis on health in the first year and an emphasis on disease in the second year. The reorganization of the course work in the first two years of the curriculum was the work of faculty in the College of Physicians and Surgeons. Ronald Drusin, the vice dean for education, Jonathan Barrasch, professor of medicine and pathology and cell biology, and Thomas Garrett, professor of medicine, planned and eliminated overlapping course content, reducing the biomedical curriculum for both the DDS and MD students from four semesters to three. A course on basic psychiatry was added back into the dental curriculum; this course had been offered during the early decades of the school's history but was subsequently eliminated.

The CDM used the shift in the biomedical sciences curriculum as an opportunity to develop an integrated preclinical dental curriculum in the freed-up fourth semester. The integrated preclinical course (see description in the "Adult Dentistry Section" in this chapter) enhances students' preparation for clinical education. They are better able to take on patient care activities in the summer following this integrated preclinical course. A series of clinical clerkships correlates behavioral and biomedical science courses in such subject areas as oral health instruction, analysis of patient-provider interactions, medical history taking, and intervention in addictive disease and nutrition analysis. Students present the medical management of their own special-needs cases in primary medicine grand rounds in the third year and discuss in small groups their comprehensive-care patients in the fourth year. As a result, the number of hours of student contact has been reduced, allowing an opportunity for an honors program in the fourth year.

The curriculum also includes two hospital rotations: a four-week rotation for experience in hospital general dentistry and a four-week

INTERPROFESSIONAL EDUCATION

Interprofessional education and practice is being encouraged at CDM and in medical centers around the country to improve the quality of health care. Essentially, such practice requires physicians, dentists, nurses, social workers, nutritionists, and others to collaborate with those in other professions and occupations that can have an impact on the outcome of patients' health. One of the new initiatives at CDM includes improving interprofessional education so that students learn the manner in which they can engage in cooperative practice.

Dr. Kavita Ahluwalia, associate professor of dental medicine at CDM, has been working with nursing and home-care staff at Isabella Geriatric Center in Upper Manhattan to improve the oral health of institutionalized older adults with dementia and community-dwelling seniors, respectively. As part of this work, Dr. Ahluwalia trained nurses to recognize and document oral health needs and to train and supervise nursing assistants to provide daily oral care. CDM has established a dental facility that is staffed by CDM faculty and dental postdoctoral students in Isabella. And in another unique partnership, Dr. Ahluwalia has teamed up with New York City's Department for the Aging and City Meals-on-Wheels to determine the oral health needs of the homebound elderly serviced by the program. Dr. Ahluwalia is finding that a very high percentage of the homebound, more than 40 percent, report difficulty in eating because of pain and oral dysfunction associated with their untreated oral disease or from ill-fitting dentures. She has developed and delivered training for social workers who visit recipients of home-delivered meals and has developed a directory of dental providers in New York City that social workers can use to link clients to dental services. She has also worked with the Department for the Aging to develop a system to document oral health needs among this population and is working to develop a home visitation program to address oral health needs in this vulnerable population.

hospital rotation to gain experience in physical diagnosis. These types of rotations have been a mainstay of the students' education for most of the past 100 years. Presently, the CDM maintains agreements with sixteen hospitals for the general dentistry experience and twelve hospitals for the physical diagnosis rotation. New York City offers a superb environment for enriching the curriculum for students because of the abundance of hospitals that accept students on rotation. In both medical and dental education, hospital rotations vary in their ability to enhance students' education from very effective to limited effectiveness. The associate dean in charge of this program, Dr. Louis Mandel, collects student comments. Of course, students' opinions on the effectiveness of the four-week rotations vary. One student's comment summarizes how these arrangements work out for students who learn a lot. This student said, "If you're not doing work here, it's because you are not volunteering to help out. There is always plenty of work for everyone, but you have to put yourself out there to get it. If you show yourself capable, expect to receive a large amount of work that can be intimidating to complete, but you can definitely do it because the residents are very encouraging and helpful."

THE SECTIONS' OFFERINGS

Adult Dentistry Section

The Section of Adult Restorative Dentistry includes two divisions, the operative dentistry division and the prosthodontics division. Dr. Richard Lichtenthal (SDOS 1962), James Winston Benfield Associate Professor, chairs the section and the operative dentistry division, while Dr. George Shelby White (DDS, NYU 1975, and Prosthodontics, SDOS 1992) is director of the division of prosthodontics. There are twenty-three faculty members in the section. The division of operative dentistry is responsible for predoctoral operative dentistry course work and the general dentistry clinical curriculum. The division also sponsors the postdoctoral advanced education in general dentistry program in which twenty-one postdoctoral students are enrolled. Of the latter students, six hold DDS or DMD degrees from U.S. dental schools and fifteen are international students from Central and South America, the Middle East, India, and Asia.

The faculty members in operative dentistry are general practitioners and coordinate the patient care program for the students. The predoctoral students are prepared for their clinical years (years three and four) through a recently reorganized core technique course. The course has been recast from individual disciplinary courses into a comprehensive care/general dentistry model, which effectively models how students

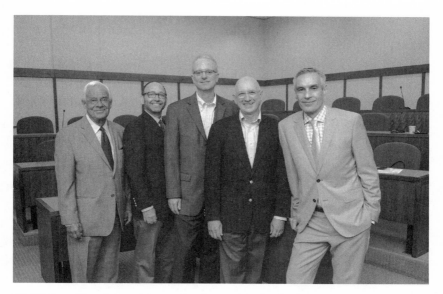

FIGURE 5.4 From left to right are the chairs of the five CDM sections: Richard Lichtenthal, Steven Chussid, Sidney Eisig, Burton Edelstein, and Panos Papapanou.

will treat and manage patients in the general dentistry clinic. This program is designed to move students through a sequence of course work taught one afternoon a week in the first three semesters and from simple to complex cases. It culminates in a fourth semester consisting of a four-day-per-week preclinical course built around a series of eight comprehensive-care cases. The reorganization of the biomedical curriculum from four to three semesters made this arrangement possible. The preclinical cases are presented with small-group discussions, each with a faculty leader. Each case requires students to present a diagnosis and treatment plan and provide treatment on a typodont that simulates the case. The students learn to use the electronic case record, as they will use this type of record when they move into the clinic. The faculty has found this type of integrated preclinical education prepares the students better for actual patient treatment than individual courses.

Regarding the clinical education program, this section has taken the responsibility to build on the comprehensive-care program begun in the 1980s (Chapter 3) and develop it into an interdisciplinary program with the general dentists taking the lead. They have appointed faculty to serve in the role as leaders of student groups and to coordinate the services of the specialists required.

The Division of Prosthodontics provides course work and faculty to teach the preclinical courses and clinical instruction in that discipline for the DDS students. In addition, the division offers a three-year master of science degree postdoctoral program for graduates who wish

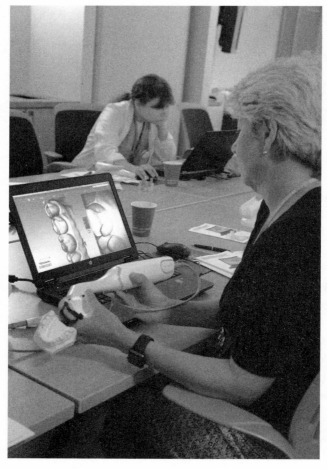

FIGURE 5.5 CAD/CAM technology is replacing older procedures used to create crowns. Patient treatment is facilitated through newer techniques. Here Dr. Jessica Hilburg (foreground), assistant professor, and Dr. Candice Zemnick, associate professor, both in the adult dentistry section, are learning how to use CAD/CAM technology.

to become board-qualified in the specialty. Four postdoctoral students are enrolled each year into the program. They graduate from a variety of dental schools at such universities as the University of Pennsylvania, Harvard University, New York University, and Rutgers University and include international students. The division is moving toward incorporating computer technology (CAD/CAM) into designing and fabricating crown restorations. Instead of taking conventional impressions of the tooth requiring a crown and sending them to a laboratory for construction of the crown, this new technology takes digital impressions via scans of the tooth and mouth and uses them to direct a milling machine to fabricate the crown.

Oral and Diagnostic Sciences Section

This section, led by Dr. Panos Papapanou (DDS, University of Athens, Greece 1984, PhD, Goteborg University, Sweden 1989, DDS, SDOS 2001) has four divisions: periodontics, endodontics, oral biology, and oral and maxillofacial (OMF) radiology, and also administers the CDM program in implant dentistry. All units provide courses to the DDS and postdoctoral students. The postdoctoral programs in periodontics and endodontics, established in 1947 and 1965, respectively, are nationally and internationally recognized. The periodontic postdoctoral program is one of the oldest programs in the United States. At the time these postdoctoral programs were first offered as specialty fields, Columbia faculty provided national leadership to organize them as specialties in dentistry.

The Division of Periodontics is planning to reorganize the DDS education using a new model of vertical integration with the postdoctoral curriculum. Third-year DDS students will join the postdoctoral periodontics curriculum in groups of five students at a time for a two-week rotation. DDS students will be paired with periodontal residents and attend their didactic and clinical sessions, which will enhance the education of graduating students significantly in this specialty area of dentistry. There are six postdoctoral residents enrolled in the three-year master of science program. The residents are truly a diverse group, coming from the United States and Europe, South America, Asia, and Australia. The division is also planning a combined four-year residency program in periodontics and prosthodontics for selected students who will have cross-training in both specialties in the fourth year. The section has submitted a doctoral program for approval to the University senate.

The research program in the division of periodontics is robust. Dr. Ulrike Schulze-Späte conducts studies on bone metabolism and osteoimmunology. Dr. Evanthia Lalla focuses her research on the identification of undiagnosed diabetes in the dental setting. Dr. Yiping Han, a recently hired microbiologist, works on the role of a common periodontal bacterial species (*Fusobacterium nucleatum*) in the pathobiology of adverse pregnancy outcomes and colorectal cancer. Dr. Panos Papapanou investigates gingival tissue transcriptomes in the pathobiology and classification of periodontitis. Dr. Papapanou also works on collaborative studies on periodontal microbiota and incident glucose intolerance and on the oral and periodontal status of an elderly cohort with various levels of cognitive impairment in the Washington Heights/Inwood Columbia Aging project (WHICAP).

The Division of Endodontics has restructured its postgraduate program, accepting six applicants per year. Each postgraduate student completes 350 endodontic cases during training along with a vigorous didactic component. Several of the graduates have moved on to academic positions throughout the world: Nova University, the University of Buffalo, Texas A&M, Baylor University, and universities in Switzerland and Saudi Arabia. The director of the division, Dr. Charles (Chuck) Solomon (DDS, SDOS 1958), and the program director of the postgraduate program, Dr. Martin (Sahng Gyoon) Kim, an endodontist who also holds an MS degree in oral biology from the University of Pennsylvania, are engaged in regenerative research on the dental pulp. Working with colleagues at the Columbia Engineering School, the division and Dr. Gunnar Hasselgren, former director of the Division of Endodontics, are developing a scaffold to permit stem cell attachment and proliferation. Research using a bioactive membrane to enhance the healing of the attachment apparatus of the tooth after an endodontic lesion has destroyed periodontal tissue is underway.

The implant program continues to grow at the Vanderbilt Clinic. In 2011 a gift of $1 million made it possible to reconstruct the Implant Center. The center provides education for predoctoral and postdoctoral students. Dr. Dennis Tarnow, a recognized international leader in dental implants, heads the Implant Center at CDM. Patients requiring dental implants have their implant surgery completed in the Implant Center by all dental specialties that provide such surgical care. A part-time (two days per week) two-year program is offered to dentists who already have specialty education (usually in prosthodontics) and wish to be trained in the surgical implant techniques. Over the period from July 1, 2011, through December 31, 2014, the school-wide implant programs have placed 6,399 implants in 2,127 patients.

The section is considering adding a new specialty program in the field of OMF radiology, which is the only specialty program recognized by the profession that is not currently available at the CDM. One of the full-time faculty members, Dr. Cleber Silva (DDS, SDOS 1998), is currently enrolled in a specialty program in OMF radiology at the University of Washington and his return will strengthen the available expertise in this field at CDM.

Hospital Dentistry Section

This section is led by Dr. Sidney Eisig (DDS, NYU 1980, and OMFS, Long Island College 1982) a board-certified oral and maxillofacial surgeon. Its offerings include DDS predoctoral courses in such subjects as OMF surgery, OMF pathology, physical diagnosis, local anesthesia, pain control, and temporomandibular joint (TMJ) and facial pain. It also offers small-group seminars for the dental students in health and disease (pathophysiology). This section is responsible for the New York–Presbyterian Hospital residency programs in OMF surgery, general practice, OMF pathology, and through the Section of Growth and Development, pediatric dentistry. The six-year residency in OMF surgery includes medical school and one year of general surgery. It is a very competitive program, with residents entering from dental schools such as Columbia, Harvard, University of Pennsylvania, McGill University, Tufts University, and University of British Columbia. As mentioned earlier in Chapter 3, the program was the seventh OMFS-MD program organized in the United States in the 1980s. Now its strengths are many and include orthognathic surgery, cleft lip/palate and craniofacial surgery, dentoalveolar surgery, outpatient anesthesia, implants, and pathology. The Division of Oral and Maxillofacial Surgery is a key member of the Craniofacial Center. The division makes at least two annual cleft lip/palate missions to Colombia, Mexico, and Guatemala. Dr. Eisig has been to Neiva, the Colombia site, at least fifteen times. At the latter site, he and his team examine and treatment-plan approximately 700 children with cleft lip and palate, microtia, and orthopedic deformities, and operate on 185 children across five days. Further, with the assistance of the speech pathology graduate outreach program at Teachers College directed by Dr. Cate Crowley, local speech pathologists have been educated on the care of cleft lip/palate patients. Orthodontic care for these patients is also arranged. In addition, there is an ongoing collaborative study with Dr. Wendy Chung, a Columbia University Medical Center (CUMC) geneticist, evaluating the etiology of clefting in Colombia.

This past year the division recruited an OMF surgeon who is fellowship trained in pediatric craniomaxillofacial surgery. The OMF surgery division is planning further expansion by recruiting an OMF surgeon with fellowship training in head and neck cancer surgery to approach such surgery on a multidisciplinary basis with other hospital services. Future plans also call for recruitment of a dentist trained in oral medicine and oncology and starting a fellowship in maxillofacial prosthetics to round out the expansion of the head and neck cancer service. Two PhDs in the division, Daniel Oh (PhD, Yeugnam University 2003) and Chang Lee (PhD, Columbia 2010), perform translational stem cell research to reconstruct skeletal and soft tissue defects. Dr. Eisig has a close collaborative relationship with Gordana Vunjak Novakovic, PhD, of the Department of Bioengineering, working with autologous stem cells and scaffolds for craniofacial regeneration. Other studies include regeneration and repair of the TMJ. Another study with Wendy Chung, MD, PhD, from the Department of Pediatrics/Division of Medical Genetics involves the identification of genetic markers in specific craniofacial/oral-facial disorders. It is hoped that this project will be translated into personalized medicine for the prognosis of congenital and developmental disorders.

The oral and maxillofacial pathology residency program is now being led by Dr. Angela J. Yoon (MPH/MAMSc, Boston University 1999, and DDS, SDOS 2003) and Dr. Elizabeth Philipone (DMD, University of Medicine and Dentistry of New Jersey 2004, and OMF Pathology, Long Island Jewish Hospital 2007), who is also a faculty member in the hospital's Irving Cancer Center. Both have NIH grants funding research into the role microRNAs play in squamous cell carcinomas. Dr. Jennifer Bassiur (DDS, University of Maryland 2002, and Orofacial Pain, UCLA 2005) directs the Center for Oral, Facial and Head Pain. Continuing a long interest in TMJ pain and its treatment at Columbia, Dr. Bassiur heads up the treatment team with patients with TMJ pain, myofascial pain, neuropathic pain, and trigeminal neuralgia—conditions that are difficult to treat. The general practice residency program rounds out the various programs of the section. The one-year program with an optional second year enrolls six hospital residents each year. Dr. Gregory Bunza (DDS, NYU 1989, and MS, Polytechnic University 1992) heads this program.

The Salivary Gland Center is directed by Dr. Louis Mandel (SDOS 1943), the last member of the faculty who graduated from the School of Dental and Oral Surgery during the World War II years (see Chapter 2). Dr. Mandel is still very active in the field in his ninth decade of life treating patients with a variety of salivary gland diseases and publishing case reports in peer-reviewed dental journals such as the *Journal of the American Dental Association*, the *Journal of Oral and Maxillofacial Surgery*, and the *New York State Dental Journal*. Dr. Mandel at one time in his long career at Columbia served as codirector of the Division of Oral Surgery and helped restore hospital operating room privileges for oral surgeons in the 1970s. He still serves as course director for the predoctoral courses in OMF surgery and the students' outside hospital rotations (see also the earlier description of the hospital rotation program for the DDS students).

Section on Population Oral Health

The Section of Population Oral Health's (SPOH) mission is to advance the oral health of populations through transformative education, research, service, and policy. This section is headed by Dr. Burton Edelstein (DDS, SUNY Buffalo 1972, and MPH, Harvard University School of Public Health and Pediatric Dentistry at Children's Hospital, Boston 1977). The mission of this section is achieved through working with a multidisciplinary team of faculty, staff, and trainees. This includes faculty and staff in such fields as pediatric and geriatric dentistry, pediatric nursing, public health, social work, sociology, and biostatistics, as well as physicians, and community health workers. For the DDS students, a full range of courses are offered in such subjects as oral health care–delivery systems, geriatric dentistry and gerontology, tobacco cessation, cariology, health promotion, dental interviewing, and narrative medicine. Unique postdoctoral opportunities are available through collaboration with the Mailman School of Public Health. Earlier dental school programs (Chapters 2 and 3) to offer joint instructions with public health have been replaced by a coordinated five-year DDS–MPH scholars program. Two students are selected annually to pursue this program, which provides them support through a federal grant. Through 2015, the program had five graduates. The program permits students to combine their clinical interests in general and pediatric dentistry, orthodontics, and prosthodontics with public health in order to advance the oral health of underserved populations. In addition, SPOH, for example, has two postdoctoral dental public health trainees engaged in the doctoral program in epidemiology at the Mailman School of Public Health. The section plans further expansion of doctoral options with the School of Public Health and behavioral nutrition.

Research activities under the direction of Burton Edelstein deal with early childhood caries intervention, an interest in the school that extends back to the early period in its history as described in Chapter 1. However, the current research aims to prevent, manage, and suppress caries in young children at high risk of dental caries through a collaborative and multidisciplinary home-intervention program. Supported by federal grants, the research team is testing the effectiveness of a culturally appropriate family-centered, home-based oral health promotion endeavor involving parents. With colleagues from the School of Nursing, the section's studies also assess the accuracy and utility of caries risk-assessment techniques and the use of culturing caries-implicated bacteria to identify the prevalence and incidence of caries experience in young children for triaging, counseling, and referral purposes. The Medicaid program is also the focus of policy studies that support such initiatives as medical-dental collaboration and promote pharmacobehavioral disease management in conjunction with dental repair. Student-mentored research has enhanced the policy agenda through investigations of dentists' and physicians' attitudes toward the Medicaid program and Medicaid beneficiaries and analyses of state practice act provisions that expand access to low-income populations.

The Community DentCare Network Program

Dr. Joseph McManus is reorganizing the Community DentCare Network program described in Chapter 3. The program has come under the umbrella of the Section on Population Oral Health. A 1972 graduate of the School of Dental Medicine at the University of Pennsylvania, McManus has extensive experience in planning and operating community-based programs. The program has operated for the past twenty-two years and provides services to the children in the Washington Heights/Inwood and Harlem communities. For most of that period, dental students in electives learned about community needs through rotations through the various sites in which the program provides care. In Washington Heights/Inwood three school clinics, I.S. 143, I.S. 52, and I.S. 164, provide prevention, basic restorative care, and emergency care to children in grades 6 through 12.

In Harlem, Community DentCare school-based clinics offer preventive dental care services in three locations at the Thurgood Marshall Academy, the Bread and Roses Integrated Arts High School, and P.S./I.S. 180/Hugo Newman College Preparatory School. These Harlem schools provide care to children in grades K through 12. Additionally, the program provides the dentists and dental hygienists to 3,000 students at the John F. Kennedy High School in the Bronx, a new endeavor in 2012 in collaboration with the New York Presbyterian Hospital. The service component is further enhanced with a two-chair mobile dental center that travels to more than eighty-two local day-care and school locations and Head Start centers throughout northern Manhattan and the Bronx. The mobile center provides comprehensive dental care to children ages three to five.

The network of community sites is unique. The program in the 2014–2015 year provided approximately 15,000 patient visits to almost 7,000 children. While many dental schools operate mobile dental vans, few, if any, operate such a school-based van program. It is unique because it brings care to the children in these sites at no cost to the parents. The dentists providing care in the sites are all members of the CDM faculty. The specialty facilities at the main site of the CDM on 168th Street in the Vanderbilt Clinic are available to provide services not available in the on-site community locations. The program has widespread community support. The vision for such a program began with Frank Thorn Van

Woert in the 1920s (Chapter 1) and was revived in the 1960s by Harold Applewhite (Chapter 2). It was finally realized in the 1980s with a widespread collaborative effort of dental faculty members and Dean Formicola with the School of Public Health, the New York Presbyterian and Harlem Hospitals, and leaders in the community and school principals (Chapter 3). The Community DentCare network was a major team effort to find a way to provide a response to a major health problem facing the community: inadequate preventive and treatment services for oral disease. The Community DentCare program received the ADEA William J. Gies Foundation award for outstanding achievement by an academic dental institution in 2014. Its reorganization as an integral part of the SPOH will strengthen the program and lead to new opportunities for students.

Section of Growth and Development

The Section of Growth and Development is under the direction of Dr. Steven Chussid (DDS, 1988 SUNY Buffalo, and Pediatric Dentistry, Women's & Children's Hospital of Buffalo 1990), who also is the director of the pediatric dentistry division. The Division of Orthodontics, directed by Dr. Sunil Wadhwa (DDS, SDOS 1996, and PhD and Orthodontics University of Connecticut 2002) is also included under this section. Both divisions provide course work for the DDS students and have postdoctoral programs in their specialty fields. From early in its history Columbia offered postdoctoral training to dentists wanting to become specialists (see Chapter 1). The predoctoral program in pediatric dentistry, under the direction of Dr. Shantanu Lal (BDS, Manipal University 1998, Pediatric Dentistry, Columbia 2001, and DDS, Columbia 2005), provides didactic and clinical instruction to the DDS students. Students also receive special instructions in recognizing child abuse. A student chapter of the American Academy of Pediatric Dentistry engages in outreach activities such as health screenings and health fairs in the community. The division also prepares students for global health externships.

The pediatric dentistry postdoctoral program is a residency program in the New York Presbyterian Hospital at the CUMC. Under the leadership of Dr. Richard Yoon (DDS, SDOS 1998, and Pediatric Dentistry, SDOS and New York Presbyterian Hospital 2001), this residency program is highly sought after—approximately 200 applications are received for the five two-year hospital positions available. Those enrolled received their dental degrees from such dental schools as the University of Connecticut, SUNY Stony Brook, New York University, the University of Pennsylvania, and Columbia. The graduates have a splendid record in passing the American Board of Pediatric Dentistry examinations, with a 100 percent success rate in both parts of the examination. The pediatric dentistry division operates a busy patient-care program located on Haven Avenue in the Allan Rosenfield School of Public Health building. Approximately 12,000 patient visits are provided annually at this facility. In addition, the residents provide consultations, emergency care, and treatment to inpatients at the Morgan-Stanley Children's Hospital at CUMC. Faculty and residents serve on the craniofacial team treating cleft lip and palate patients and other special patients such as transplant and hematology/oncology patients. The division cooperates with ongoing research in the Section on Population Oral Health described above (the early childhood caries intervention family-centered program).

The orthodontic division provides course work to the DDS students and graduate dentists. The orthodontic postdoctoral program led by Dr. Jing Chen (DDS, Peking University 1994, 2006 PhD, University of Connecticut 2006, Orthodontics, University of Connecticut 2011, and DDS, CDM 2013) continues Columbia's long tradition in this field. The three-year program enrolls seven new students each year who have graduated from such schools as Harvard, Medical University of South Carolina, the University of Toronto, the University of Karachi, and King Saud University. Each of the incoming first-year postdoctoral students takes on approximately sixty to seventy-five new cases and treats them throughout the three-year program. All of the postdoctoral students are required to submit and defend a research thesis to earn the master of science degree. There is an active research program, two major studies of which aim to study the TMJ and how it is affected by occlusal loading and estrogen receptors. Bone and cartilage during development, disease, and regeneration are areas of investigation in the orthodontic research laboratory. The orthodontic alumni association is an active group that holds regular meetings for graduates. For example, they hosted a spring meeting named for Dr. Thomas Cangialosi (DDS, Georgetown 1959, and Orthodontics, SDOS 1975), the former long-term director of the division of orthodontics and Leuman M. Waugh Professor of Clinical

Orthodontics (Emeritus). Dr. Cangialosi is now Professor and Chairman of the Department of Orthodontics at the Rutgers University School of Dental Medicine.

THE RESEARCH PROGRAMS OF THE COLLEGE OF DENTAL MEDICINE

The College's founders, among them William J. Gies, PhD, urged dental schools to pursue research in order to understand oral disease and treat it better. Today the research efforts of the CDM faculty are vigorous. Supported by funds from the NIH and other government and private sources, faculty members are pursuing research in six programmatic areas, including (1) oropharyngeal cancer; (2) biomaterials/regenerative biology and stem cells; (3) neuroscience and pain; (4) microbial pathogenesis/microbiome; (5) behavioral sciences/health sciences; and (6) systemic and oral disease interactions. These studies over the seven-year period of 2009 through 2015 have been supported by approximately $43 million in outside federal and nonfederal grants, on average about $6.2 million per year and almost $7 million in 2015. The faculty involves both predoctoral and postdoctoral students in their studies. Over the same period of time, 185 predoctoral students and seventy-six postdoctoral students joined research efforts. Each year beginning in the 1950s, the College celebrates the research accomplishments of its students and its faculty mentors in the Birnberg Research Day program. A lecture by a noted researcher is followed by student poster presentations, some of which are selected for awards. Dr. Carol Kunzel (PhD, NYU 1979) is director of research at the college. Her descriptions of research grants received and studies underway, compiled from NIH Web-based sources and information from the investigators, have been included in the previous section descriptions and in Appendix 4, which contains details of the six program areas conducted by the faculty.

FUTURE PLANS FOR THE COLLEGE OF DENTAL MEDICINE

By the start of the 2015–2016 year, Christian Stohler had held several faculty retreats to continue discussions on the findings from the strategic planning efforts and to discuss future directions. While some of his specific plans and those of the section heads were described earlier, there are several major key initiatives that could solve a variety of long-term issues for the CDM and strengthen it for the future.

One of the plans includes gaining additional space for the College, a long-term issue recognized since the very first move of the school to the Vanderbilt Clinic in 1928 (Chapters 1–3). While additional space for the College was gained in the last three decades of the twentieth century, another contiguous floor in the Vanderbilt building has been long sought. An opportunity was missed during the deanship of Gilbert Smith when the school failed to annex any of the additional floors that were added to the Vanderbilt Clinic above the three floors dedicated to the dental school. However, the floor below the dental school space, VC 5, has now been made available to the dental school, and the dean has hired a consulting firm to decide the best use of this additional floor to relieve the crowding on the three existing floors. This additional floor will be a major step forward for dentistry within the CUMC and the University. The design of this additional floor is to be unique and will incorporate all of the latest computer technology enhancing the educational and service programs. Additionally, plans to include the west side of Presbyterian Hospital seventh floor will provide the CDM with a greater presence within CUMC.

A second major advance the dean and the faculty are planning is to reconceptualize the off-site educational and service initiatives at CDM. Such programs would fit into three categories: urban, rural, and global. Plans call for enhancing the urban initiative under the Community DentCare program (described in Chapter 3 and earlier in this chapter) through reorganization and a new site in Manhattanville (part of west Harlem), a site where Columbia University is expanding its Morningside campus. At Manhattanville, the dean, working with University officials, is considering establishing an off-site dental clinic. The new clinic would service patients in that neighborhood, which is bordered by 133rd and 125th Streets north and south and Broadway and the Hudson River east and west. This plan would be a major expansion of the College's ability to provide care to the underserved populations in northern Manhattan. In 2016 the first new University building to be completed on this site, just north of the main campus, is the Jerome L. Green Science Center, which will house the Mortimer B. Zuckerman Mind, Brain, Behavior Institute. A dental clinic would be a major benefit to the residents in the nearby neighborhood and would fit into the University's commitment to enhance the environment for those living nearby.

Government reports indicate that one of the most serious shortages of physicians and dentists is in rural America. In addition to the expansion in the urban network, the CDM is considering a new initiative in rural oral health care. In 2010 the College of Physicians and Surgeons began an innovative program at its affiliated Bassett Medical Center in the rural community of Cooperstown, New York. A cadre of ten to fifteen students spend their clinical clerkship year of medical school in the Bassett health system, which provides them the opportunity to experience rural medicine at both the individual patient and population level. As the CDM explores its future options for its students through its strategic planning process, it is examining whether the Bassett Medical Center program presents a similar opportunity for dental students who would spend their last clinical year in the underserved area. Using distance learning and telemedicine, dental students could remain in contact with the faculty at the 168th Street site while spending their final year in Cooperstown, New York, and engaging in clinical practice within the Bassett health system. Dr. Ronnie Myers, vice dean for administration, is working to explore this option with Dr. Stephen Nicholas, associate dean for admissions at P&S, and Dr. Henry Weil, assistant dean for education at Bassett Healthcare, as well as others at the Bassett Medical Center and other interested parties responsible for the P&S program.

The College of Dental Medicine is planning to continue the global health externship program in which more than 40 percent of its students participate. Established during the first decade of the twenty-first century (see Chapter 4), the children's global health initiative is a partnership with P&S and Columbia University. It is an initiative that leads teams of faculty and students to provide services in underserved countries such as Guatemala, the Dominican Republic, Cambodia, and the Philippines. Students can also participate in underserved communities in the United States through the Indian Health Service. CDM faculty and residents accompany the students on these trips, which are sponsored by service organizations such as Kids International Dental Services, Somos Amigos, and the Indian Health Service to provide necessary oral

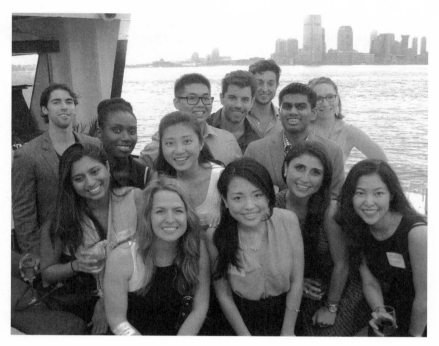

FIGURE 5.6 The alumni association always includes students at their events. Here, dental students are enjoying the Manhattan Boat Cruise alumni event.

care to these underserved areas. A total of more than 2,500 patients are seen annually on these missions.

To realign programs and keep the College of Dental Medicine in the forefront of dental education nationally and internationally, Dean Stohler is enlisting members of the board of advisors to help review plans and point the College toward the next level. While the board of advisors has helped advise the previous deans since it was established in the 1980s, this new role will provide the leadership of the College with objective input to help make the shift from the present to the future. Chaired by Leslie (Les) Seldin (DDS, SDOS 1966), a leader in national and state dentistry, the board of advisors is a diverse group of individuals that includes alumni members with wide experience in practice, academia, research, and business (see Appendix 5 for a list of the board's members). Their dedication to the CDM will make a difference in adjusting the College's mission to the rapid pace of the twenty-first century.

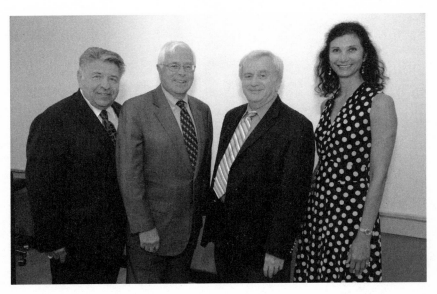

FIGURE 5.7 Task force leaders of the board of advisors are (from left to right): Steven Kess, Leslie Seldin (chair of the board of advisors), James Lipton, and Madeline Monaco. Appendix 5 lists all of the members of the board of advisors.

In Chapter 1, Houghton Holiday, the associate dean from 1935 to 1946, unwittingly used just the right words to conclude this chapter. As he reflected on the development of the profession during the first three decades of the twentieth century, he was aware that times were changing. He said, "There are changing and growing demands being made upon the profession which must be reflected in the teaching program . . . It is very easy to be tied down to the past, accepting what is, as what should be. We need to tear ourselves loose from tradition and periodically, if not constantly, readjust our profession to the changes which are taking place."[3] Dean Stohler has become dean at the College of Dental Medicine at a similar time of change. His administration will point the College into the second 100 years and keep the CDM continually moving to become "a dental school on university lines" as envisioned in the founding document.

CHAPTER SIX

Students and Alumni

The founding document, *A Dental School on University Lines*, set out a goal for the Columbia University Dental School, as it was first called, to have high standards in selecting students for enrollment. It recognized that students studying for careers in medicine and dentistry should be prepared similarly in college for their joint studies in the biomedical sciences in the first two years of professional schools. In selecting students to enroll, SDOS/CDM has been vigilant in making sure that those who study at the CDM have the academic preparation and ability to be successful in the highly regarded joint medical/dental instruction in the first two years. In addition, in selecting students the school has looked for applicants with wide interests. Over the past 100 years, the "school on university lines" has drawn a talented student body, many of whom have become leaders in the field and dedicated alumni. These graduates have excelled in many arenas: private practice, academia and research, and in leadership positions in professional organizations and public health. We have already shared some of those graduates' stories in earlier chapters. We share others in this chapter and include a focus group discussion with students enrolled during the 2014–2015 academic year when the book was being written.

THE STUDENT BODY

As noted, the College of Dental Medicine has always attracted a talented and well-prepared student body. For example, in the dean's report of

June 30, 1939, Dean Rappleye noted that only fifty out of 315 applicants were selected. Even at that time, students were selected from the top of the applicant pool, and the demographics show that they attended twenty-two different colleges and universities.

The dental school has a long history of accepting a diverse group of students. When Columbia merged with the College of Dental and Oral Surgery (CDOS) in 1923, it inherited a large, robust, and diverse student body. For example, 14 percent of the students in the class of 1919 were women. In 1993, then Dean Formicola spoke with Dr. Henrietta Ofner, one of the thirty-two women in that class and a distinguished New York City practitioner. Ofner explained that when Columbia and other dental schools decided to require two years of college as a prerequisite for entrance, it became difficult for most women to continue to qualify for admissions. In fact, as a result of the new requirement for at least two years of college preparation, most women were squeezed out of the profession. However, the students in the class of 1922, who were enrolled prior to the new requirement, were able to attain a graduation rate of 11 percent women. In Dr. Ofner's case, she entered CDOS after graduating from Washington Irving High School and, like most women at that time, was not encouraged to attend college.

As the new requirement for at least two years of college preparation (first set by Columbia) became accepted across the nation, dentistry became a male-dominated profession. The Depression years and World War II created further obstacles to women being able to enter dental school. A scan of the SDOS graduating classes from yearbooks and student enrollment records showed that in 1922, in the pre-Depression and prewar years, 11 percent of the graduates were women; but in a subsequent forty-year period, between 1932 and 1972, only four women graduated! It was not until the social revolution and the women's movement in the 1960s and the 1970s that the country reawakened to the idea that the medical professions should be opened to all people regardless of race or gender. Things began to change then, and by 1982, 18 percent of SDOS graduates were women. The School of Dental and Oral Surgery continued to attract increasing numbers of women to its DDS classes. Forty-nine percent of the entering class in the seventy-fifth anniversary year (1990–1991) was composed of women, exceeding their 39 percent representation in the national applicant pool.[1] Today the College of

Dental Medicine enrolls almost equal numbers of men and women, with 46 percent of the class of 2018 being women.

African American graduates followed a trajectory similar to that of female graduates. SDOS and its predecessor institution, CDOS, always admitted a few African American students. For example, there were two male African American students among the 1922 graduates from CDOS. In 1923 Anna Elizabeth (Bessie) Delany (1891–1995) graduated from CDOS. She was African American and a resident of Harlem. During the Depression, Dr. Delany provided free dental care to residents of Harlem

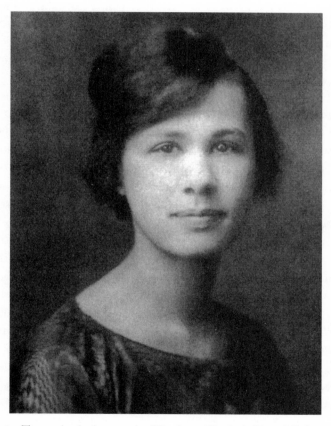

FIGURE 6.1 The yearbook photograph of Dr. Anna Elizabeth (Bessie) Delany, a graduate of SDOS in 1923. The coauthor of the best-selling book, *Having Our Say*, with her sister, Sarah (Sadie) Delany, a graduate from Teachers College, Bessie speaks about her time at SDOS in the book.

in her private office. She would become famous later for coauthoring the acclaimed book *Having Our Say* with her sister, Sarah (Sadie) Delany (1889–1999). A graduate of Teachers College, Sadie Delany earned a master of education degree in 1925.

Having Our Say became a best seller and was made into a Broadway play and a television movie in 1995 and 1999, respectively. Both sisters were in their 100th year of life when they wrote the book reflecting on life in New York City. Bessie Delany described some of her experiences at Columbia: "My brother Harry was a dentist, and he was going to see if I could enroll at New York University, where he had graduated. But this was in 1918, and New York University would not take women in its dentistry program. Instead, I enrolled at Columbia University . . . in the fall of 1919. There were eleven women out of a class of about 170. There were about six colored men. And then there was me. I was the only colored woman!"

In the book, Dr. Delaney also described some incidents at the school that made her feel that there was discriminatory treatment of her as an African American student. "To be fair—oh, it's so hard to be fair— I have to admit that some of them (faculty members) treated me just fine, especially the Dean of Students. He was an old white man, yet he was particularly supportive of me. But one instructor really had it out for me. There was an assignment where he failed me, yet I knew my work was good. One of my white girlfriends said, 'Bessie, let me turn in your work as if it was mine, and see what grade he gives it.' I'll tell you what happened, honey. She passed with my failed work! That was the kind of thing that could make you crazy, as a Negro." Here at age 100-plus years old she still vividly recalled this type of treatment, which was endemic of how students of color, if they were even accepted, could expect to be treated, except at historically black dental schools, until the social revolution in the 1960s and 1970s.[2]

The number of African American and Hispanic students has fluctuated over the past 100 years at the SDOS. Beginning in the 1980s and 1990s and well into the new century, the School of Dental and Oral Surgery made efforts to attract underrepresented minority students to its applicant pool and placed major emphasis on being more welcoming to underrepresented minority students. Dr. Albert Thompson, an African American alumnus of the school, has been a longtime advocate for the recruitment of minority students. While a student at Columbia College, he was a star athlete on Columbia's track and field team. He held championships in the shot put and discus and qualified for the 1956 U.S. Olympic trials. After graduating from Columbia College in 1954 and serving in the U.S. Navy, Thompson returned to Columbia and graduated from SDOS in 1960. He became a part-time member of the faculty and served as a member of the admissions committee and as the chair of the committee on minority affairs. That committee considered many of the issues necessary for the school to open its admissions process to minority students.

The school next conducted a climate study to improve the environment for the recruitment of underrepresented minority dental students. Dr. Marlene Klyvert (BS, 1971, MS, 1972, MEd, 1977, and EdD, 1980, all at Columbia), a graduate of the dental hygiene program and full-time member of the faculty, took on the responsibility to oversee the implementation of the recommendations from the climate study. She provided guidance to the school's executive committee on how to improve the atmosphere as recommended by the climate study.

The postdoctoral specialty program with Harlem Hospital began in 1988, as described in Chapter 3. That program educated twenty-three underrepresented minority general practice dental residents at Harlem Hospital in the dental specialties and in public health at the Columbia University Medical Center and provided the opportunity to further SDOS's efforts in this direction. Several of the graduates became either full- or part-time faculty members at SDOS, expanding what had been a small cadre of longtime minority faculty members. Dr. Michael Bolden was the first of the Harlem Hospital residents who completed the specialty program in periodontics. This program helped SDOS make further advances in the recruitment of minority applicants for the DDS program as several of the graduates joined the full- and part-time faculty.

Dr. Dennis Mitchell (DDS, Howard University 1989, and MPH, Columbia 1996), one of the Harlem Hospital residents, enrolled in the MPH program at the Mailman School of Public Health, joined the full-time faculty in the dental school upon completion of the program. With the assistance of longtime faculty members Drs. Marlene Klyvert and Albert Thompson and with the encouragement of the faculty and administration of the school, Mitchell helped to enhance the climate to attract a critical mass of underrepresented minority students.

Dr. Mitchell was instrumental in obtaining a grant from the Robert Wood Johnson Foundation for a summertime academic-enrichment program aimed at assisting underrepresented minority college students and others to prepare themselves for careers in medicine and dentistry. He became a mentor to underrepresented minority students aspiring to a career in dentistry. As a result of his and the school's efforts, 20 percent of the students in the class enrolled in the fall of 2014 were underrepresented minority students. Through the efforts of the school and reflecting the accomplishments of the underrepresented minority students who enrolled during the 1990s and the first decade of the twenty-first century, the College of Dental Medicine was awarded a prestigious HEED (Higher Education Excellence in Diversity) award in 2014. The award is given to institutions that demonstrate outstanding commitment to diversity and inclusion. The CDM was the first dental school in the nation to be recognized with a HEED award. In 2014, Dr. Dennis Mitchell, senior associate dean for diversity affairs at the CDM, was selected to become the Columbia University vice provost for faculty diversity and inclusion. Mitchell stated that for the CDM to achieve being a destination for the world's greatest scholars "requires that diversity be a fundamental core value of inclusion and excellence and it be evident in recruiting, advancement, retention and experience." Chapters 3 and 4 also have more information on the diversity program.

As a result of these efforts, by the fall of 1991, eight, or 11.4 percent, of the seventy entering students were African American, and three, or 4.2 percent, of the students were Hispanic. The school also attracted a large group of Asian/Pacific Islander students; 45 percent of the entering class in 1991 was from this population group. The classes as a whole continued to be selected from the top 10 percent of the applicant pool based on the Dental Aptitude Test scores. Today, the class of 2017, the centennial class, is 20 percent underrepresented minorities, 48 percent male, and 52 percent female. The students in this class came from fifty-three different colleges, and twelve states. Class size has grown steadily over the years. By 1960 the class size was sixty incoming students, and by 2017 the incoming class size was eighty. There were 2,266 applicants to CDM from the 11,719 national applicants. While the students entering CDM are diverse and come from many different colleges and states, from time to time local students from northern

Manhattan apply and enroll. One of those individuals in the class of 1981 was Dr. Rosa Martinez.

ACHIEVING HER DREAM: ROSA MARTINEZ (DDS, SDOS 1981)

Dr. Rosa Martinez grew up on West 103rd Street, a stone's throw from the Columbia University Morningside campus. She completed her pre-dental studies at City University. She says, "Columbia was my dream school. It was the only institution that my parents talked about when I was growing up. One of their aspirations was that one day one of their daughters would be able to attend and obtain a degree from Columbia University." And Rosa did just that by entering SDOS and graduating in 1981 with her DDS degree. Of her education at SDOS, Dr. Martinez stated that the basic science education was second to none and "Dr. Mel Moss [former dean and professor of anatomy] was larger than life and his anatomy course was excellent." Her Columbia education, with its strong emphasis on systemic health, has guided her during her career. She has built this educational approach into the general practice residency program she heads at the Westchester Medical Center, where she also serves as the director of dental services and holds a faculty appointment at the New York Medical College. Reflecting back on her twenty-eight-year career, Rosa said that she valued the education she received at Columbia and "always strives to represent the CDM well by doing the best that I can to make my past professors proud." Her alma mater is proud of her!

EXPANDING STUDENT VOICES

New York City is a city built on immigrants and a diverse group of people of all races, creeds, and ethnicities. The College of Dental Medicine and its predecessor institutions strove to reflect the city in which the school resides. While the mix of students has resulted in an energetic student body, it was through the improved relationship between the school and its student body that its graduates became more involved and contributed to the alumni association. Up until the late 1960s and 1970s, students felt they had relatively minimal voice in how dental schools were operated and that few administrators sought their opinions in how to improve the educational environment. Then, after the student protests in the 1960s and 1970s, attitudes of the faculty and administration toward college and professional students began to change across the nation and at SDOS.

One of the goals of the school during the 1980s was to become more inclusive in its operation and to treat students as junior colleagues. The school recognized that its students were mature young men and women who had already completed college. Many even held master's degrees. As such they could add immensely to the academic environment. Those who chose to attend school at Columbia did so because of its strong academic reputation; in fact, most Columbia students were accepted at five or six other dental schools but made Columbia their first choice. And one of the students was even a fireman!

A CIRCUITOUS ROUTE: GEORGE SHEEHAN (DDS, SDOS 1982)

Dr. George Sheehan exemplifies the scope of life experiences some students bring to SDOS. Sheehan's own tenacity and determination played no little part as he followed a circuitous route to SDOS, entering the school ten years after graduating from high school and a stint in the infantry in Vietnam. He completed his predoctoral education at three different colleges before earning his BA in Sociology at Queens College.

He decided to pursue going to dental school because he "liked working with my hands and did well in the sciences. I enjoy people, and dentistry came out of that thought process." Sheehan, who graduated in 1982, credits Dr. Stan Brzustowicz (DDS, 1943) a full-time faculty member, for motivating him. After Sheehan's admission interview Brzustowicz said, "I am betting on you, don't let me down." Sheehan applied to dental school while a New York City firefighter attached full-time to Ladder Company 34, located at 161 Street between Broadway and Amsterdam Avenue. He remained with that firehouse during his four years of dental school. He was married with one child when he entered SDOS in 1978; his daughter was born in 1980. His wife and the firemen he worked with made it possible, he said, for him to be able to be successful in the challenging dental school curriculum while being

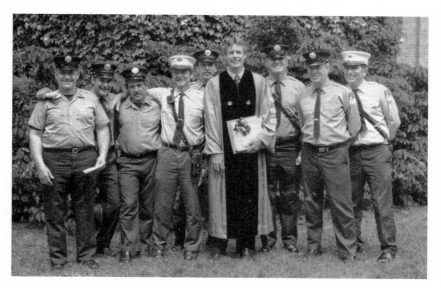

FIGURE 6.2 While a student at SDOS, George Sheehan also held down a full-time position as a firefighter. He is shown here with his colleagues from Ladder Company 34. The fire trucks parked on Fort Washington Avenue and sounded their sirens for George during the 1982 graduation ceremony in the Garden!

a full-time fireman. In fact, Ladder Company 34 was so proud of him that when he walked across the stage to receive his diploma, firemen lined the walkway and fire trucks sounded their sirens and horns! Today, George is a successful general practitioner in Garden City, New York.

* * *

Students were given a voice at Columbia. They were appointed to committees such as the curriculum committee and the ethics committee. The position of dean for student affairs was expanded from a half-time position to a full-time one to improve services for students. Dr. Martin Davis (DDS, SDOS 1974, and Pediatric Dentistry, 1975) the director of pediatric dentistry, moved from his leadership position in pediatric dentistry into the position of assistant dean for student affairs. Davis set about to codify the school's various academic policies by creating a new extensive document called the *Academic Policies and Procedures Manual.* The manual served to clarify student promotion policies and student due process rights. He established a daily "walk-in hour" at which students could obtain advice on all matters. Another important tradition was begun to bring the students more closely into the affairs of the college—a monthly luncheon meeting for the student government officers and class presidents and the dean and the student affairs dean. Open discussion of any issues affecting individual classes or the student body at large was conducted during this lunch meeting. All of this contributed to student attitudes toward their school changing in a positive direction.

Today dental students have a well-organized student government and group of activities in which they participate. At the College of Dental Medicine, an associate dean supports many of the student and alumni activities. Among these are an orientation program for the incoming freshman students; the Academic Success program, a peer tutorial program for first-year students; and a variety of student chapters of national organizations.

STUDENT RESEARCH

The dental school offers an active student research program. Approximately 25 percent of the second-year students are engaged in research working in laboratories in basic science, dentistry, medicine, public health, and engineering. A number of the student activities are embedded in the culture of the institution and reach back to the early years of the school's formation.

The William Jarvie Society, organized on December 16, 1920, is one of those student-operated organizations. William J. Gies, with William Jarvie as its benefactor, organized it. The purpose of the society was to promote the spirit of research among students, a concept that was so forward thinking at the time that the minutes of the William Jarvie Society's first meeting were published in the *Journal of Dental Research*. While the society has waxed and waned in its activities over the past century, it has flourished over the last forty years. In 1989 the *Journal of the William Jarvie Society* began again to publish its annual journal as announced by its then editor, Dr. Vincent Ziccardi (DDS, SDOS 1989), who went on to earn combined oral and maxillofacial surgery training and an MD degree at Columbia. He is now chair of oral and maxillofacial surgery at the Rutgers University School of Dental Medicine in Newark, New Jersey. The history of the society has been carried forward through the annual publication of the *Journal of the William Jarvie Society*. The organization and the journal are student run with faculty advisors.

The alumni association of the School of Dental and Oral Surgery established a research award in the early 1950s to further encourage student research. The award is named in honor of Dr. Frederick Birnberg (1893–1968), a member of the class of 1915 who helped to establish a research fund at the school. The recipients of the Birnberg Award are national experts and become visiting professors who participate in Research Day activities. The visiting professor presents a lecture at the dental school on Research Day, a day that highlights student research at the school. Student table clinics and research posters are presented on the day of the lecture. Together the Jarvie Society, the *Journal of the William Jarvie Society*, and the Birnberg Award/Research Day activities highlight student research by DDS students and postdoctoral students.

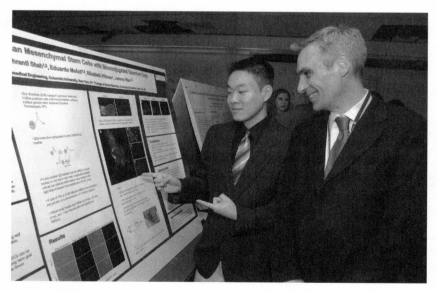

FIGURE 6.3 Dr. Panos Papapanou, chair of the Section on Oral and Diagnostic Sciences and director of the Division of Periodontics (right), discusses the findings of a dental student at the student poster session during Birnberg Research Day.

Dr. Jeffery Hajibandeh (DDS, CDM 2014), student president of the Jarvie Society, wrote in the *Journal of the William Jarvie Society* in 2014, "The William Jarvie Research Society has played a vital role in stimulating student interest in research and scientific discovery."[3] There were fifty-eight student members of the society, demonstrating the depth of the student body's interest in research. The scope of the students' interest is obvious from the presentations on Research Day in 2013. There were twenty-five predoctoral presentations and seventeen postdoctoral presentations given on April 9, 2013.

Papers ranged from "Multiphase Bioscaffold for Integrated Regeneration of Root Periodontium Complex" to the "Inter-relationships Among the Oral Complications of Diabetes Mellitus" and from "Alveolar Bone Changes to Orthodontics in an Osteopenic Patient with Possible Hajdu-Cheney Syndrome" to "Caries Risk Assessment Utilization by Pediatric and General Dentists." Both William Gies and William Jarvie would be thrilled that eighty years after its founding, the society continues to encourage a spirit of research in the student body. Clearly the tradition established early on by the founders to encourage a spirit of research and inquiry in the student body is still alive, 100 years after the founding of the school. An energetic and talented student body begets an energetic and talented alumni body. Opportunities are many at Columbia, and faculty encourage students to pursue their interests. Dr. James Lipton took advantage of available opportunities and was encouraged to pursue his interests.

JARVIE SOCIETY MEMBER: JAMES LIPTON (DDS, SDOS 1971, AND PHD, GRADUATE SCHOOL OF ARTS AND SCIENCES 1980)

James Lipton was a member of the Jarvie Society when he was a student at SDOS. When asked about the strengths of his dental education, he says, "The major strength of my Columbia education was being at Columbia. It was exciting." He also cited the basic science courses with medical students, being able to do research in the medical school, the opportunity to take several courses at the graduate school on the Morningside campus, and "the strong personal support provided by most of the clinical faculty" among his positive experiences. Lipton credits

Dr. Robert Gottsegen with supporting his interest in public health and the social sciences. It was Gottsegen who encouraged him to enroll in the School of Public Health for the PhD program, which he completed in 1980. Lipton says that he was able "to take advantage of the wonderful opportunities provided at this great institution." He certainly has used his Columbia education well: He has had a distinguished career in both the U.S. Public Health Service and the National Institute of Dental and Craniofacial Research. Upon retiring from the Public Health Service, Lipton became an adjunct professor at the University of Pennsylvania School of Dental Medicine. Dr. Lipton has served on the CDM Board of Advisors for more than ten years.

POSTDOCTORAL TRAINING

From the very inception of the dental school, its faculty recognized the need for graduates to continue their education with postdoctoral training. Strong postdoctoral training programs were at the core of the school's founding when it incorporated the New York Post-graduate School into the dental school in 1917. While dentistry does not require a period of postdoctoral training for licensure to practice, Columbia's dental school encourages all students to seek residencies in hospital programs or in postgraduate specialty programs. And graduates heed the recommendation.

For example, the class of 2013 had 95 percent of its seventy-seven graduates move on to postdoctoral training. They had an enviable record in being accepted into premier postdoctoral programs in the dental specialties and in general dentistry. Seven of the graduates were accepted into oral and maxillofacial surgery programs, seven into orthodontic programs, and five into pediatric dentistry programs, while another eight were accepted into periodontic, endodontic, prosthodontic, or oral radiology programs. Thirty-four of the graduates were accepted into hospital residencies or dental school general dentistry programs. There are not a sufficient number of postdoctoral training slots for all of the graduates from the nation's dental schools. So such a high degree of acceptance of Columbia's dental school graduates is a sign that its graduates are heavily recruited by postdoctoral training program directors.

Many of these graduates and others point to faculty mentors who influenced their careers. A few examples: Ronald Dubner (DDS, SDOS 1958), who also earned a PhD in physiology, is an international expert on the neurobiology of pain and conducted his research career first at the National Institutes of Health and then at the University of Maryland. When asked by *Primus* who inspired his first interest in this topic, he said: "I was also influenced by one of my SDOS professors, Dr. Laszlo Schwartz, a pioneer in studying temporomandibular pain and its relationship to neural mechanisms in the trigeminal regions."[4]

Paul Baer (DDS, SDOS 1945, and Periodontics, SDOS 1955), when asked why he chose Columbia for dental school, said the following: "Well, there were only two places to go for dental education in New York City, and at the first one I visited the faculty and students were using foot pedals to power their instruments! When I got up to Columbia, I found they were using electricity. Columbia also offered the advantage of small classes where I got more time with my instructors, one of whom was Dr. Frank Beube, a major influence on me and in my chosen field."[5] Baer went on to become a major researcher and educator in the field of periodontics at the State University of New York, Stony Brook, School of Dental Medicine.

Dana Graves (DDS, MS, SDOS 1980), when asked by *Primus* how he discovered that dentistry would eventually lead him to research, responded, "It was probably at Columbia when Dr. Irwin Mandel assigned me to do a follow-up on a European study of immunoglobulins in saliva. I couldn't reproduce the original study's results and feared I'd made errors in my work. But, it turned out I was right and the study was wrong."[6] Graves has distinguished himself in research and as chair of the Department of Periodontics at the University of Pennsylvania School of Dental Medicine.

Columbia attracts graduates of other dental schools to its postdoctoral specialty programs. Many devote their careers to full-time specialty practices. These graduates also point to the important role of faculty mentors in their education. Dr. David Goldberg points that out in reflecting on his experiences at SDOS.

FACULTY MENTEE: DAVID GOLDBERG (DMD, RUTGERS UNIVERSITY SCHOOL OF DENTAL MEDICINE 1979, AND PERIODONTICS, SDOS 1982)

In looking back at his postdoctoral education, David Goldberg said he "was blessed to receive an incredible education" at SDOS. Goldberg, a board-certified periodontist, was a DMD graduate from nearby Rutgers University School of Dental Medicine when he chose to come to Columbia for his postdoctoral training. Columbia stood out because he realized that many of the giants and authors in the field of periodontics were at Columbia. He saw that the strengths of the program included the diversity in the periodontal faculty members who were experts and authors in a broad range of methods from conservative therapy to surgical approaches to treat peridodontal disease. This solid educational foundation has helped Dr. Goldberg springboard into much more complex implant and regenerative surgeries he now uses routinely.

In addition, Goldberg points out, the College of Dental Medicine is located in New York City. This location draws visiting faculty from around the world and "they would come to Columbia." Jan Lindhe, Cliff Ochsenbein, and Saul Schluger, three giants in the field of periodontics at the time Dr. Goldberg attended, were some of the individuals who he and his postdoctoral colleagues were exposed to.

While studying in his chosen field at SDOS, Goldberg was impressed that there were opportunities to engage in research along with distinguished faculty. He cites Dr. Daniel Fine, a longtime faculty member at SDOS and now at the Rutgers University School of Dental Medicine, as one of the faculty members to include him as a member of his research team. Goldberg is a successful private practitioner in North Plainfield, New Jersey, whom *New Jersey Monthly* magazine selected as a "Jersey Choice: Top Dentists" since 2002. He said that he was "proud of my Columbia education, proud of the fine reputation of the school, which is going in the right direction." In fact, Goldberg was also happy that his son, Adam, selected the CDM to attend and has successfully completed his freshman year at the time this book was being written.

THE ALUMNI ASSOCIATION AND ALUMNI RELATIONS

The Association of Dental Alumni of the SDOS was formed in 1923. It was established as a component of the Columbia University Alumni Federation, which was formed in 1895. Until the incorporation of the CDOS into Columbia's Dental School, there were fewer than fifty Columbia graduates. But the freestanding CDOS had approximately 2,000 graduates by the time of the merger. In 1940, a special committee of the alumni association decided that the graduates of the College of Dental and Oral Surgery should join the ranks of the Columbia alumni. The special committee noted in its report to the University that both the law school and the medical school had incorporated the alumni of the predecessor schools that merged with them.

As the SDOS Alumni Association grew, it supported events that reflected the academic focus of the school. For example, in 1949 the association sponsored a caries symposium featuring leaders in the field such as Dr. Joseph Volker. Volker was dean of the Tufts Dental School in Boston and later president of the University of Alabama at Birmingham. On the twenty-fifth anniversary of SDOS, 250 dental alumni attended a luncheon in Bard Hall featuring Dr. Basil Bibby, a renowned leader in dental research. Over the years the alumni association established several awards, which are still presented today, including the Fred Birnberg Annual Research Award described earlier and multiple awards presented to deserving seniors at the May graduation ceremony.

By 1985 the association was a robust organization, hosting a number of events, some of which continue today, including the fall picnic at Baker Field and the annual alumni reception at the Greater New York Dental Meeting. The association engages with the student body, inviting them to all events and giving them tokens of appreciation and recognition throughout the year. They have recently created a formal mentoring program, matching third-year students with alumni and faculty mentors.

It is fitting to include in the 100-year history of the College of Dental Medicine, the names of the presidents of the alumni organization. They are listed in Appendix 6. Margot Jaffe, who served as president of the alumni association from 2008 to 2011, is a good example of an SDOS alumna who greatly appreciated her education at Columbia. Her story mirrors that of the other alumni who give back to the college through service after receiving the benefits of its educational opportunities.

GIVING BACK: MARGOT JAFFE (DDS, 1980, PEDIATRIC DENTISTRY, 1981, ORTHODONTICS, 1985, ALL AT SDOS)

Margot Jaffe was raised in Queens, New York, and received a BS in biology at Trinity College in 1976. She applied to four dental schools in the Northeast—and was admitted to all of them. However, she says she selected Columbia "because of the strong medical basic science, its location and because it was an 'Ivy.'" She points out that she really "graduated three times earning the DDS in 1980, and a certificate in Pediatric Dentistry in 1981 through a special honors program, and then again in 1985 with a certificate in orthodontics." The honors program combined the senior year in dental school with the first year in post-doctoral training and was an innovative program in the 1970s and early 1980s. Thirty students completed the program before it was terminated due to accrediting agency objections.

Jaffe currently has a full-time private practice in pediatric dentistry and orthodontics in Manhattan. She is also an assistant clinical professor in pediatric dentistry at the College of Dental Medicine, a post she has held for thirty years. Additionally she sits on the admissions committee, is a past president of the alumni association, and presently sits on the dean's board of advisors. She is also the district I trustee of the College of Diplomats of the American Board of Pediatric Dentistry.

Choosing "an Ivy" was a good decision for her. She feels that her Columbia education helped her in her career path in that "I received an excellent education both didactically and clinically," thanks to "a fantastic basic science curriculum, world renowned faculty and small class size, and many mentors who instilled in me a 'quest for excellence.' Dr. Martin Davis was a special mentor—a terrific selfless educator, an advocate for all children, a motivator, and very active in organized dentistry on the local and national level."

In addition, she says, "All my jobs as an associate were obtained through school networking and faculty who vouched for me. I have had the benefit of wonderful patient referrals, and help from faculty on developing a private practice. I was recommended to sit on committees at the American Academy of Pediatric Dentistry early on in my career and have maintained a very active role in the academy."

Jaffe says that in a sense, her thirty-five years at the CDM have never been interrupted. "I have developed lifelong friendships, tried to uphold all the ethical principles that were taught to me, and have tried very hard to give back and mentor students. In other words, I have a stake in perpetuating the excellent education and promoting professional relationships in the current student body." Margot's son, Keith Goldman, is currently (at the time this book was being written) in his second year of the orthodontic postdoctoral program.

The importance of networking and the high regard for Columbia University held by the public is another attribute of studying at Columbia according to Jose Fossas, a postdoctoral graduate from the orthodontic program. He expresses such sentiments in his story. Fossas followed in his father's and grandfather's footprints, coming from Puerto Rico to study at Columbia.

FAMILY FOOTPRINTS: JOSE FOSSAS (ORTHODONTICS, 1994)

What could make a stronger statement about the quality of a school's educational experience than to have the children of alumni study there? Such is the case with the Fossas family. Three generations of the Fossas, who originated in Puerto Rico, have attended Columbia. Dr. Arturo Fossas earned a certificate in orthodontics in 1957 and his son Jose came to Columbia for his postdoctoral work, completing his orthodontic training in 1994. Jose said, "Being the son of a Columbia orthodontist and grandson of an alumnus of the Columbia School of Engineering, I made my decision without any hesitation [to attend the orthodontic program at Columbia]." Fossas says he appreciated the program for the diversity of orthodontic techniques taught at Columbia. He notes that most other programs emphasize only one or two techniques. He feels that his professors were enthusiastic teachers and outstanding in their respective fields. Drs. Lawrence Seigel, Melvyn Leifert, and Malcolm Mistrel are names that "always come to mind" in the latter category. Fassas says, "It is an honor to be recognized as a Columbia alumni," as it is always mentioned when he meets other professional people and there is value in being part of the Columbia network. While Fassas was enrolled in the program, his father came to visit the school from their home in Puerto Rico. Fassas was amazed that after almost forty years, his father was recognized right away by one of his faculty members, Dr. Julius Tarshis! Fossas also cited Columbia's "worldwide reputation as an excellent academic institution" as another reason for wanting to study at SDOS. Jose Fossas, who is currently in private practice, says, "The memories of the good times are endless."

Specialty Alumni Organizations

Graduates of the postdoctoral specialty programs, whether they are undergraduates of the Columbia DDS program or have completed their dental degree at another university, are proud of having attended one of the specialty programs. The periodontic and orthodontic programs have set up independent alumni organizations, and regular networking events are organized for the alumni of these programs and for the programs in pediatric dentistry, oral and maxillofacial surgery, prosthodontics, and endodontics. In the 1990s the alumni from the various specialty programs raised sufficient funds to reconstruct the specialty clinics on the Vanderbilt Clinic ninth floor. Their efforts made it possible to reconstruct the facilities with modern equipment for orthodontics, periodontics, endodontics, and prosthodontics.

The dental hygiene alumni continued to be active in the field and involved with CDM despite their program having been discontinued in the 1980s due to low enrollment. The alumni association established an annual Patricia McLean (1906–1983) Dental Hygiene Symposium in memory of the director of the program who served between 1964 and 1977. Her son, John McLean (DDS, 1965 and Orthodontics, 1972, both at SDOS), and other alumni, friends, and family members provided a generous grant to help establish the symposium. The annual symposium attracts many CDM dental hygiene alumni as well as dental hygiene practitioners from the region. The topics are contemporary issues in dental hygiene. For example, the 2014 symposium was "Peri-Implant Maintenance: An Evidence-Based Approach." McLean was very active in dental hygiene organizations, having served as president of the Dental Hygienists Association of New York City and chair of the Council of Auxiliaries of the American Association of Dental Schools. She was held in high esteem by her students and the faculty and was well known nationally. In addition to her role as director of dental hygiene, she was also appointed assistant dean of SDOS by Dean Zegarelli in the late 1970s.

In 1990 a full-time position was created at the school to enhance alumni affairs. Melissa Welsh serves as director of alumni relations and continuing education. She is the liaison between the alumni association and the school and also implements schoolwide, regional, national, and international events for alumni. Welsh also helps to develop publications and programs designed to strengthen alumni ties with the school and its faculty and students and with the broader University community. She works closely with Geraldine Connors, director of development, who is responsible for the school's fund-raising efforts. Over time, the fund-raising activities have enlisted thousands of the school's alumni/ae to assist it to meet its mission and goals.

FUND-RAISING AT THE SCHOOL OF DENTAL AND ORAL SURGERY

The alumni association, in conjunction with SDOS, agreed in 1979 to eliminate the membership fees. Since then, all graduates automatically become members of the alumni association, with the school supporting the majority of costs of the alumni events and carrying out professional fund-raising efforts. The goal of this action was to encourage all of the alumni/ae to become active in school/college events and support their alma mater.

The Annual Fund

The school started an annual fund in 1980 to establish a strong base of alumni contributors. More than $90,000 was raised in the inaugural year, helping to make up for increasing cutbacks in federal and state aid. Since that time, the annual fund has supported scholarships for talented students to study at Columbia regardless of their ability to pay and for other projects and programs.

In 1982 Dr. Irving Naidorf (DDS, SDOS 1942) the assistant dean for postdoctoral programs at that time served as chair of the school's first annual fund drive for major donors. He worked with the alumni association to form the 1852 Society, an organization that recognizes the highest level of annual giving by alumni and friends. Members of the society made a minimum yearly commitment of $1,000 to the annual fund. The 1852 Society is so named to honor the year of establishment of the New York College of Dental Surgery, the earliest antecedent of SDOS. Dr. Eugene LaSota (DDS, SDOS 1961) was the first chair of the society and was followed in order by Dr. Susan Karabin (DDS, SDOS 1981, Periodontics, 1984), Dr. Thomas Connolly (DDS, 1977, Perio, 1980, both at SDOS), Dr. Daniel Zedeker (DDS, SDOS 1983), and Dr. Thomas Magnani (DDS, SDOS 1980), the current chair. Success with the annual fund helped in establishing successful capital fund-raising campaigns in the 1980s and 1990s.

The Capital Campaign

Capital fund-raising was a low priority at the medical center up until the 1970s when the Medi Center 1 Capital Campaign was established. It was the first fund-raising effort at the medical center that included all four Columbia University health science schools and the Presbyterian Hospital, and was instituted to aid construction projects and build endowment support. The SDOS campaign concluded in December 1980, with $6.6 million raised for the reconstruction of dental facilities and special projects and an additional $2 million raised toward the school's endowment. Dr. Joseph Leavitt (DDS, SDOS 1941), founding director of the Division of Endodontics and a successful practitioner, oversaw the dental school's fund-raising efforts throughout the 1970s and early 1980s. Dr. John Lucca (DDS, SDOS 1947), director of the Division of Prosthodontics, was enlisted as chair for the second five-year (1987–1992) capital campaign, the seventy-fifth anniversary campaign. And Dr. Susan Karabin (DDS, SDOS 1981 and Periodontics 1984) chaired the third five-year (1992–1997) Pathways to the Future campaign. Through their hard work and the generosity of alumni and other donors, the school raised $15 million for renovating many of the facilities on the seventh, eighth, and ninth floors of the Vanderbilt Clinic and for endowment and special programs. In 2005 a new capital campaign was undertaken by Dean Lamster (Chapter 4) with Dr. Thomas Connolly (DDS, SDOS 1977 and Periodontics 1980) serving as chair. By 2010 this campaign had raised an additional $21 million for renovation of facilities, endowment, and special programs, and by December 31, 2013, the end of the campaign, a total of $26.2 million was raised, surpassing the original goal for the campaign by $11.2 million. Dr. Thomas Magnani (DDS, SDOS 1980) has agreed to serve as the next campaign chair for the College of Dental Medicine's major centennial campaign.

Both Dr. Irving Naidorf and Dr. Joseph Leavitt were deceased when this book was written. However, in addition to their leadership in fund-raising, both were close colleagues and left their imprint on the Division of Endodontics. As pointed out earlier in this book, they were leaders in the formation of endodontics as a recognized specialty field in

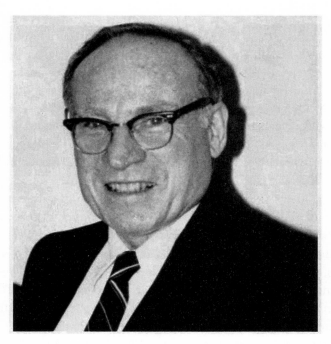

FIGURE 6.4 Dr. Irving Naidorf (DDS, SDOS 1942) served as a long-time faculty member in the Division of Endodontics and as assistant dean for postdoctoral programs. He was the first chair of the 1852 Society, the annual fund-raising program.

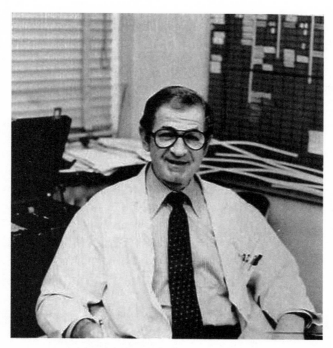

FIGURE 6.5   Dr. Joseph Leavitt (DDS, SDOS 1941) served as the chair of the first SDOS Medi Center 1 Capital Campaign in the 1970s. He, along with colleague Irving Naidorf, was an early pioneer in developing the specialty of Endodontics. Leavitt founded the Division of Endodontics at SDOS.

dentistry in the 1960s. Leavitt was also the founding director of the Division of Endodontics at Columbia. The legacy of their collaboration was still evident in comments from a 1993 DDS graduate from the University of Minnesota, Dr. Tom Pagonis, who completed the endodontic post-doctoral certificate program at Columbia. Pagonis, who holds a part-time faculty appointment at the Harvard School of Dental Medicine, said that the "synergy of research, intellectual curiosity and clinical care" were the important hallmarks of the Columbia program, traits Naidorf and Leavitt handed down to their successors in the Division of Endodontics. As Dr. Pagonis put it, Dr. Gunnar Hasselgren, a leader in the endodontics division when he was studying at Columbia, followed in his predecessors' footsteps by being a "tremendous influence as a mentor who instilled intellectual curiosity, research and professionalism."

Such comments reflect the heritage of these two leaders who joined the faculty from the School of Dental and Oral Surgery classes in the 1940s.

RECOGNIZING DISTINGUISHED ALUMNI

University Recognition

Beginning in 1933, the Columbia University Alumni Federation (now the Columbia Alumni Association) annually recognized alumni for distinguished service of ten years or more to the University, including its schools, alumni associations, or regional Columbia clubs. The thirty-five graduates of the SDOS/CDM who have been so recognized are listed in Appendix 7. Dr. Thomas Connolly received the Alumni Medal in 2015, the year this book was written.

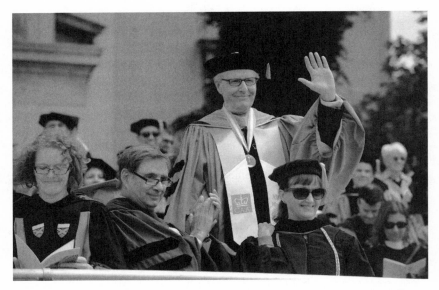

FIGURE 6.6 Dr. Thomas Connolly (DDS 1977, Periodontics 1980, both at SDOS) received the Alumni Federation Medal for Service to the College of Dental Medicine at the 2015 Columbia University commencement. He is wearing the medal. Dr. Lee Goldman, the executive vice president and dean of the Faculties of Health Sciences and Medicine and chief executive of the Columbia University Medical Center, applauds him for his contributions.

In addition to alumni who have been honored by the Columbia Alumni Association, three honorary degrees have been awarded by Columbia University to SDOS faculty, one in 1929 to Alfred Owre, the dean from 1928 to 1933; a second in 1983 to Edward Zegarelli, the dean from 1973 to 1978; and the third to Irwin Mandel in 1996.

School of Dental and Oral Surgery/College of Dental Medicine Recognition

The graduates of the College of Dental Medicine have achieved notable accomplishments in the field of dental medicine. Many have distinguished themselves in academia, in research, in practice, or in service to the school or to the profession. The College is justly proud of all of its graduates. Beginning in 1990 the School of Dental and Oral Surgery began to recognize graduates with the Distinguished Alumni Award. Twenty-four such awards have been made through 2013. They are cited in Appendix 8 chronologically in the years awards were received.

Many other graduates have distinguished themselves in the profession, some in leadership positions in organized dentistry, while others have made major contributions in academia and research. A snapshot of some of those who have distinguished themselves are listed in Appendix 9. Over the past 100 years, the College of Dental Medicine has contributed much to the profession and in service to the public. For all those recognized by the University or the school/College, there are hundreds of others who have not been recognized. Those cited in this book through stories or those listed in the appendixes are just examples of the many Columbia University College of Dental Medicine graduates who have gone on to serve the public and the profession. The unrecognized alumni, however, have been recognized in their home cities or schools where they practice or teach as Columbia graduates who uphold high standards. There is no better recognition than that.

It is fitting that the last chapter of this 100-year history is devoted to students and alumni/ae. The very purpose of educational institutions is to provide the proper environment to educate the next generation of citizens. Health professional schools have a special obligation in preparing practitioners and scientists for the good of the public. The history of this school depicts the various stages it went through to achieve that purpose. It shows that it is not easy to have high standards and continually achieve them. However, when looking back over the past 100 years of history of the Columbia University College of Dental Medicine, it is apparent that the school continually strove for excellence to meet the high bar set by being a school within Columbia University. The graduates of the School of Dental and Oral Surgery, now known as the College of Dental Medicine, reflect the founders' vision through their careers in the field of dentistry and their service to the public.

Throughout the book stories of alumni were included. Their stories illustrated various points regarding the dental school. As the College of Dental Medicine begins its next 100 years, the voices of the current students, the next generation of practitioners, researchers, public health workers, and faculty, need to be heard. In June of 2015, Allan J. Formicola, dean emeritus, sat down with a group of enrolled students to listen to their thoughts on studying at the College of Dental Medicine.

WHAT THE STUDENTS SAY

Members of the student body can provide an insight into the current environment of the College of Dental Medicine. To capture that insight, the author of this book met with a group of enrolled students in a focus group arrangement. Eight students, six enrolled in the DDS program and two in the postdoctoral program, attended. Students in the DDS program were in the second, third, and fourth years of the program, and the postdoctoral students were second-year students in periodontics and orthodontics.[7] Four of these students were from New York, two from Florida, and two from New Jersey. They attended various colleges and completed a diverse set of majors. Those colleges included University of South Carolina; SUNY Stony Brook; Rensselaer Polytechnic Institute; University of California, Berkeley; Cornell University; University of Miami; Duke University; Carnegie Mellon University; and Trinity College. Their undergraduate majors included finance, mechanical engineering, pharmacology, French, economics, chemistry, and biological sciences. The postdoctoral students earned their DDS degrees from University of Pennsylvania School of Dental Medicine and Columbia University College of Dental Medicine. They brought to the CDM a diverse educational background, which bodes well for the future of the College and the profession. What follows are their responses to a series of questions about their experiences at the CDM and their views on the future of the College and the profession.

The Environment for Students at the College of Dental Medicine

When asked why they selected Columbia for dental education, the prevailing view was, as one student put it, because "the college is in New York City, the school is a top school, the pass/fail grading system, a special 'something' about the student-faculty relationship, and a warm and welcoming atmosphere." All agreed with these statements and added that they all had had a wide choice of schools at which they were accepted (and "some were less costly"). However, these attributes of the CDM made it a desirable place to study. The group stated that the admission process reflected the school positively. The interview process was pleasant, and meeting with enrolled students over lunch provided them with a positive view of the school—a view that held up once enrolled. They pointed to the school's alumni as mentors who were considerate of the difficult course load they carried. For example, they cited Dr. Lois Jackson (DDS 1977, and Pediatric Dentistiry, 1980, both at SDOS), who "brought ice cream for all of the students during an intense exam period, which relieved the tension they were under." Also they pointed to Dr. Thomas Magnani (DDS, SDOS 1980), who "stayed until late in the evening to work with students in the preclinical laboratory, helping [and] advising them on technique course work." The students felt the faculty were similarly supportive. The postdoctoral students recognized their programs as being supportive of a variety of opinions and taught by knowledgeable faculty members who were authors of papers and textbooks. One of the students said, "At the end of the day, there are great people here that make up the College of Dental Medicine family." The students credited Dr. Laureen Zubiaurre Bitzer (DMD, Fairleigh Dickinson 1996), associate dean for admissions and student affairs, and Sandra Garcia, assistant dean for admissions and student affairs, for fostering this atmosphere.

Comments on the Curriculum

Regarding the curriculum, the students appreciated the quality of the medical school basic science course work in which they were enrolled.

They believed that the depth of this course work gave them an "edge up" in relation to other dental school graduates. One student said that it was appropriate that the dental students had the "same foundation in the medical sciences as do the medical students because dentistry is as much of a medical specialty as are other medical specialties." Another student agreed but wished there was a little more balance between the basic science curriculum and the clinical curriculum. The group realized that the dental science courses were undergoing a difficult transition to incorporate technology. One student pointed out that the current generation of students is entering professional school from colleges that are incorporating a personalized approach to education with online courses, which allow students to learn at their own speed. This was the wave of the future and dental schools would need to get there too. The students recognized that the dean, Christian Stohler, was addressing technology in education. They cited the school's adoption of the use of CAD/CAM technology in restorative dentistry as a sign of this direction.

The Pass/Fail System of Grading

The students believed that the pass/fail system of grading was responsible for helping to create an atmosphere of cooperation between classmates and lessen the competition for grades. While they understood that postdoctoral program directors were having difficulty in evaluating the standing of graduates on the pass/fail system for their programs, they further understood that this trend would continue, as the National Board Exams dental students must take are now graded on a pass/fail system. The group was aware that the postdoctoral programs would probably require an entrance exam such as the Graduate Record Exam for admissions as another way to evaluate the pool of candidates.

Dual-Degree Program Opportunities

Students believed one of the strengths of the College was the dual-degree program opportunity. They expect that the future of dental practice will require practitioners better educated in business as group practices with multiple locations grow. They are happy those opportunities exist at Columbia. One of the students was considering the dual DDS–MBA program and two of the students are pursuing a combined DDS–master's degree program with Teachers College. They indicated that several of their classmates were enrolled in the dual DDS–MPH program and that each year two to three students graduate with those dual degrees.

Diversity Initiative

All the students in the group were positive about the College's diversity initiative and the fact that they were going to school with a diverse student body. They were pleased with the program that Dr. Dennis Mitchell runs as the associate dean for diversity and inclusion and said that diverse students allowed them to learn much about different cultures. One student explained that she was from a small town that had no diversity and went to a college where there also was little diversity. "I really didn't know about others until I came to CDM. I have learned a lot here and am glad I have the opportunity to understand the different perspectives of students different than me."

The Future

When asked about where the College and the profession were headed, the students appeared to have their sights well focused. They recognized that interprofessional education was a trend that was beneficial to patients and it was emerging and needed to be fostered more in the profession and the College. They expected that advanced dental hygienists and the practice of dental therapy would expand their ability to treat more patients and make their practices more efficient. Regarding the changes in the allied workforce, they cited medicine's adoption of nurse practitioners and physician assistants and indicated that dentistry needed to catch up with that trend. They felt that more collaborative practice modes would require teamwork and that group practices would grow. They expected the reimbursement model for dental care would change. They felt that the use of technology in practice would continue to grow and that CDM should reflect these trends too. In short, this generation of students seemed to embrace change and not be fearful of it.

Finally, one student summed up the College of Dental Medicine and the discussion by saying that the College "has smart people who are kind and compassionate people."

There is no better way to conclude the book than with the voices of those who will be the next leaders in the profession. The College of Dental Medicine is fortunate to be part of a great University located in the City of New York. The setting attracts a talented and enthusiastic student body, future graduates who will keep the profession strong while serving the public.

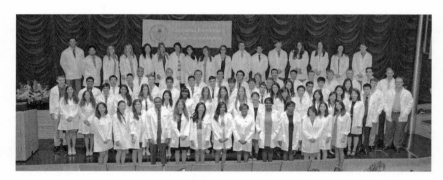

FIGURE 6.7 In 1993 Dr. Arnold Gold, a faculty member at P&S, began the White Coat Ceremony for medical students. Later, dental schools adopted a similar ceremony to welcome dental students to the profession upon their enrollment. The centennial class, the class of 2017, is shown during their White Coat Ceremony upon entering CDM in 2013.

Appendix 1

The Founding Document

Columbia University
in the City of New York

A DENTAL SCHOOL
ON UNIVERSITY LINES

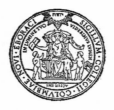

Columbia University
in the City of New York

MAY, 1916

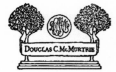
DOUGLAS C. McMURTRIE

A DENTAL SCHOOL ON UNIVERSITY LINES

Dentistry and Dental Education are on the threshold of extraordinary development but are unable to take advantage of their opportunities because of the traditional separation of dentistry and medicine.

Dentistry has been shown by recent investigations and research to be logically a branch of general medicine, and to be an increasingly important factor in the understanding, diagnosis and treatment of numerous diseases which hitherto have been obscure in origin but which are now known to arise from conditions of the mouth and teeth and can accordingly be controlled and prevented. Chronic rheumatism, anaemia, hardening of the arteries, digestive disorders, diseases of the heart and kidneys, nervous affections, neuralgia, etc., are found to be influenced and often caused by neglected mouths. It is the expressed belief of prominent physicians that the next great step in preventive medicine must come through dentistry, and that no single division in the whole range of hygiene is more important to the public than the hygiene of the mouth.

In the face of these facts, dental education finds itself in an embarrassing position because of its separation from medical education. A large majority of the dental schools of this country are proprietary institutions without medical school or university affiliations. It is obvious that a professional school, managed so as to pay a profit to its owners, cannot give to its students the advantages afforded by a professional school conducted as a part of a university at the expense of endowment funds provided by philanthropy in the interests of public service. The tuition paid by medical students is considerably less than half the cost of their instruction, and the same would be true of dental students, were their education conducted along university lines in connection with advanced instruction, investigation and research. These and similar considerations have prompted the leading dentists and physicians of New York to undertake to establish a school of dentistry in affiliation and co-ordination with an existing school of medicine. It has seemed best to propose to connect the new school of dentistry with the proposed new medical centre, to be established by Columbia University and the Presbyterian Hospital as soon as sufficient funds to finance the project are obtained.

The Trustees and the Faculty of medicine of Columbia University have, by formal vote, approved the establishment of a school of dentistry as soon as the funds for its maintenance can be obtained. It is proposed to make the dental course at Columbia one of four years, the first two years of which are to be identical with, and part of, the medical course. The preliminary educational requirements are to be the same as those for admission to the medical school. A dental dispensary, providing free treatment to the poor, opportunities for clinical experience for the students as a basis for scientific research will be one of the large features of the new school. Another important feature will be special research in dental science. Many of the problems in dental pathology can be solved only by the most careful and painstaking investigation, and upon their solution will depend, in no small measure, the health and well-being of humanity. With the first two years of a medical course as a foundation, the increased clinical material, bedside instruction in hospital wards and the greatly enlarged laboratory facilities which the new school will provide will all make for better and more scientifically trained dentists.

The proposed school has the approval of the New York Academy of Medicine, the County Medical Society, the

[4]

First District Dental Society and has the endorsement of the Health Commissioner and well known physicians and dentists, as shown by the subjoined letters and names.

A fund of $1,000,000, yielding an annual income of about $50,000 will be required to found and to maintain the proposed dental school. The undersigned express the hope that the plan to create a new and superior factor in dental education and research will merit widespread public approval and that contributions in sufficient amount may speedily become available for the effective establishment of the Columbia University Dental School.

Contributions to this fund should be made payable to the Treasurer of Columbia University and may be forwarded to him direct at 63 Wall Street, New York, or to any member of the Dental Committee named on page 7.

FINANCIAL NEEDS

Proposed Equipment

Operative department	$15,000.00
Prosthetic department	5,000.00
Oral surgery department	1,500.00
X-ray department	1,500.00
Orthodontia department	1,000.00

Proposed Operative Expenses

Rental of building unless $25,000 for brick construction on present Medical School is provided	$4,000.00
Dean and Professors of operative dentistry, prosthetic dentistry, oral surgery and orthodontia	17,000.00
Assistant Professors of operative dentistry, prosthetic dentistry, oral surgery and orthodontia	6,000.00
Instructors and chiefs of clinic	4,500.00
Infirmary staff, materials, light and heat	10,000.00
Making a total of	$41,500.00

COMMITTEE FOR
COLUMBIA UNIVERSITY DENTAL SCHOOL

MEDICAL COMMITTEE

From Medical School, College of Physicians and Surgeons

Dean Samuel W. Lambert   Dr. William J. Gies
Dr. George E. Brewer   Dr. Herman Von W. Schulte

DENTAL COMMITTEE

Dr. Henry S. Dunning, *Chairman*
Dr. Arthur Merritt, *Secretary*
Dr. Bissell B. Palmer, Jr., *Treasurer*

Dr. Leuman M. Waugh   Dr. Charles F. Ash
Dr. Newell S. Jenkins   Dr. James W. Taylor
Dr. Henry W. Gillett   Dr. William D. Tracy
Dr. Harold S. Vaughan   Dr. William B. Dunning
Dr. Frederick K. Kemple   Dr. James F. Hasbrouck
Dr. Oscar J. Chase, Jr.   Dr. William Jarvie
                Dr. Rodney Ottolengui

FROM THE MINUTES
OF THE FACULTY OF MEDICINE,
COLUMBIA UNIVERSITY
November 15, 1915

RESOLVED: That the faculty approve the foundation of a school of dentistry, if adequate funds be provided, upon university lines. The first two years should be the same as those for the degree of M.D., and with the same entrance requirements, with a special faculty, and the committee recommends that a special committee be appointed to formulate further the plans.

FROM THE MINUTE OF THE TRUSTEES
March 6, 1916

By a School of Dentistry on university lines is meant a school the requirements for admission to which shall be the same as those for admission to the Medical School and whose students shall then pursue a four-year course, the first two years of which will be almost identical with the first two years of the course in Medicine. The two last years would be given to special preparation for dentistry and dental surgery.

The Committee recommend the adoption of the following resolution:

RESOLVED: That the recommendations of the Faculty of Medicine, made at the stated meeting of December 21, 1915, and concurred in by the University Council at the stated meeting of February 15, 1916, be approved as to first, third, fourth and fifth resolutions of recommendation (numbered a, c, d and e).

The resolution was adopted.

[8]

Appendix 2

The Predecessor Institutions from 1852 Through 1923

Chapter 1 describes the history of how the Columbia University Dental School was formed. Through the 1923 merger with the College of Dental and Oral Surgery, an independent school, the Columbia University Dental School traces its history back to 1852 and a dental school chartered and operated for a short time in Syracuse, New York. The Syracuse school was named the New York College of Dental Surgery and was the first dental college in New York State and the fifth to be established in the United States. Amos Westcott was the founder and dean of the Syracuse School, which was destroyed by fire in 1856. The charter for the Syracuse school was moved to a New York City school headed by John Reed. In 1904 the charter passed to the College of Dental and Oral Surgery headed by William Carr, which then merged with the Columbia University Dental School.

It is important to record the history back to 1852. A description by Michael Kurtz of the importance of the New York College of Dentistry to the formation of the Columbia Dental School clearly shows the pathway to Columbia.[1] Under the title "Columbia University and Those Who

---

1. Michael Kurtz became interested in the history of dentistry while a student in the class of 1977. He did a masterful piece of research on the history of the formation of the dental school at Columbia. His paper, published in the October 1978 issue of the *Bulletin of the History of Dentistry*, was a winner in the 1977 Bremner Essay Award Competition conducted by the American Academy of the History of Dentistry. M. Kurtz, "Columbia University and Those Who Made It the Mecca of Dental Education," *Bulletin of the History of Dentistry* 26, no. 2 (1978):86–103.

Made It the Mecca of Dental Education," Kurtz ably describes the ties between the New York Dental School, the College of Dental and Oral Surgery, and the Columbia University Dental School:

> In 1879 the charter [of the Syracuse School] was amended "on paper" to allow the college to hold property up to $100,000. The name was thus changed to the New York State College of Dental Surgery and its location from Syracuse to New York City."

Some years later, on June 8, 1892, Dr. John Howard Reed secured the charter to establish the New York Dental School. He had graduated from the New York College of Dentistry in 1881 (founded in 1865; now the New York University College of Dentistry). Reed's New York Dental School first opened its doors on Monday, October 2, 1893, in the Kennedy Building at 289 Fourth Avenue in New York City. By 1899 all departments were moved to 216 West Forty-Second Street.

Family pressure forced Reed to withdraw from active participation in the New York Dental School in 1895. He always remained its silent partner, however, and clandestinely hoped his creation would someday be taken over as the dental school of Columbia University. Just prior to his death on March 12, 1940, at the age of eighty-one, Reed wrote to Dr. Manuel M. Maslansky:

> I was impelled about this time [1890] . . . to go forward with an urge for better things, to a definite fixed purpose of organizing a better dental school that should have a four year course . . . that should receive women on an equality with men, and that should receive students to matriculate according to the highest standards of Harvard and Ann Arbor Universities, . . . a school that should be more directly under the supervision of the Regents of New York State, and ultimately to be taken over by Columbia University as its Dental School.

In a letter written in 1892, others express a parallel desire. This document was furnished to Dr. L. Laszlo Schwartz by Charles Francis Bodecker, whose father was a signatory.

We the undersigned dental practitioners are desirous of having a dental department established in connection with the College of Physicians and Surgeons of Columbia University . . . It is our wish and intent that the students of the dental department shall study anatomy, physiology, and chemistry with the medical students of the College of Physicians and Surgeons.

It is the aim of the undersigned to create a dental department the standard of which shall be very high.

Very respectfully submitted,
Carl F. W. Bodecker, Benjamin Lord, Charles E. Francis, William Carr

William Carr, the last signatory, did in fact pick up where John Howard Reed left off. In 1904, Dr. Carr, armed with Westcott's revived charter, effectively assumed leadership of the New York Dental School under its new composite name of the New York College of Dental and Oral Surgery. In 1905, because of protests that the new corporate name too closely resembled that of the New York College of Dentistry, the name was again changed to the College of Dental and Oral Surgery of New York. The College thrived and by 1913 was moved to new quarters on Thirty-Fifth Street.

In summary, the current College of Dental Medicine dates itself back to the 1852 Syracuse school, the New York College of Dental Surgery, and then in 1892 to the New York Dental School located in New York City. In 1904 the New York Dental School became the College of Dental and Oral Surgery, which then merged with the Columbia University Dental School in 1923 to become the School of Dental and Oral Surgery. The leadership went respectively from Amos Westcott to John Reed to William Carr, who joined the Columbia faculty upon the merger.

Appendix 3

Letter from Victor S. Koussow to Arthur T. Rowe

October 28, 1935

Dr. Arthur T. Rowe
Dental School
Columbia Univ.

   From the very beginning of my work in the Dental School you permanently exercised prejudice and unjusitice toword me.
   During the Word War I was an Army Officer and I saw horrible pictures. But in peaceful civil life I never met so much cruelty such a permanent torture as I saw it from you all four years of my work here.
   Toword me all four years you were acting as a real executioner.
   Now you get results of your work.

Victor S. Koussow

Appendix 4

Funded Research Studies in the 2014–2015 Year

As discussed in Chapter 5, the College of Dental Medicine reported there were six programmatic areas of research ongoing in the 2014–2015 academic year. They were categorized under the following titles: (1) oropharyngeal cancer; (2) biomaterials/regenerative biology and stem cells; (3) neuroscience and pain; (4) microbial pathogenesis/microbiome; (5) behavioral sciences/health sciences; and (6) systemic and oral disease interactions. What follows are specific descriptions of the studies under each category prepared by Dr. Carol Kunzel, Director, Office of Research Administration at CDM.

OROPHARYNGEAL CANCER

Angela Yoon, MicroRNA Marker-based Prognosis of
Oral Cancer Survival

About half of those diagnosed with oral cancer will die of the disease within five years, resulting in more than 8,000 deaths annually in the United States. This is partially due to lack of a mechanism to predict which cancer patients may or may not fare well following the initial surgery, which is crucial in deciding the subsequent treatment procedure. Dr. Yoon's team is working to find a reliable clinical test that may identify those with poor prognosis so that additional treatment can be rendered to improve the overall cancer survival rate. [Funded by the National Institutes of Health/National Institute of Dental and Craniofacial Research (NIH/NIDCR).]

Elizabeth Philipone, Predictive Value of MicroRNAs in the Progression of Oral Leukoplakias

Oral leukoplakias or white patches are found in 3 percent of the population and approximately one-third of leukoplakias will progress to oral squamous cell carcinoma (OSCC). Dr. Philipone is working to develop a predictive clinical modality that can accurately identify progressive lesions among clinical leukoplakias. Early identification and management of progressive leukoplakias will significantly contribute to eradication of OSCC. [Funded by the National Institute of Dental and Craniofacial Research (NIDCR).]

BIOMATERIALS/REGENERATIVE BIOLOGY/STEM CELLS

Jeremy Mao, Meniscus Regeneration by Endogenous Stem/Progenitor Cells

Jeremy Mao's research laboratory has been pursuing multidisciplinary investigations in tissue engineering and stem cell biology for nearly two decades. His team reported in *Lancet* that the entire articular surface of a synovial joint condyle in skeletally mature rabbits was regenerated by the recruitment of host endogenous cells and without cell transplantation. Extending this concept to meniscus regeneration, the team found in a large animal model (pigs) that endogenous cells not only were homed but also differentiated into fibrochondrocytes by two spatiotemporally delivered growth factors. The meniscus, a wedge-shaped tissue in the knee between the thigh bone and leg bone, serves as an indispensable cushion without which the bones do not fit. Meniscus trauma is a common injury and increases the risk of arthritis. [Funded by the National Institute of Arthritis and Musculoskeletal and Skin Diseases (NIAMS).]

Jeremy Mao, Preclinical Models of Odontic Analogs by Endogenous Stem Cells

Oral diseases negatively affect one's self-esteem and impair multiple physiological functions, including mastication, digestion, and/or speech. This multidisciplinary, translational research project aims to develop ways to address the current shortage of regenerative dental devices. In the study's abstract, Dr. Mao reports: "Remarkably, host endogenous cells can be homed into anatomically correct, porous scaffolds responsible for regeneration without cell transplantation. This discovery is a continuation of broad efforts by my laboratory and many other laboratories with an ultimate goal to regenerate teeth for clinical applications." The study focuses on the regeneration of tooth roots, rather than the entire tooth, by cell homing, in a preclinical, large animal model that represents an obligatory step in the regulatory pathway. [Funded by the National Institute of Dental and Craniofacial Research (NIDCR).]

Chang Hun Lee, Roles of Perivascular Stem/Progenitor Cells in Tendon Healing and Pathology

Chang Hun Lee is studying tendon injuries, which are a significant healthcare burden given the lack of a regenerative therapy. Studies in this proposal are anticipated to reveal specific roles of a novel population of tendon stem/progenitor cells in tendon healing and pathology. The expected outcome of the proposed studies will serve as an important foundation to develop a new treatment for tendon injury and disease by harnessing endogenous stem/progenitor cells. A recent study has shown a novel strategy to regenerate tendons by harnessing a specific population of endogenous tendon stem cells.

Daniel Oh, Three-Dimensional Alveolar Bone Reconstruction and Regeneration Using a Novel Anatomically Conforming Microenvironment Scaffold

Daniel Oh has developed a bone-like microenvironment scaffold that has a fully interconnected porous structure similar to trabecular bone, as well as microchannels and nanopores, which foster the infusion of the scaffold with the patient's own bone marrow and growth factors. In terms of tissue engineering, Dr. Oh's research focuses on optimizing scaffold designs so that they are highly compatible to in vivo environments for proper cell and growth factor ingression and retention, and ultimately bone regeneration. Such studies have the potential to assist surgeons in correcting craniomaxillofacial skeletal deformities, including defects of the maxillary and mandibular dental alveolus, frequently a reconstructive challenge for both the surgeon and the patient.

Mildred Embree, DENTIST SCIENTIST K99/R00: Improve Temporomandibular Joint Fibrocartilage Regeneration Strategies

Mildred Embree is interested in ways to regenerate diseased or damaged temporomandibular joint (TMJ) fibrocartilage. Her studies propose the development of tissue-engineering strategies for biological TMJ condyle substitutes, and these studies are anticipated to be critical for the development of regenerative treatments for patients suffering from TMJ disease or injury. Through a training award, Dr. Embree aspires to obtain extensive understanding of TMJ biology and regeneration and to develop new expertise in the fields of tissue engineering and stem cell biology in relation to TMJ disease, as she progresses toward an independent dentist-scientist. [Funded by the National Institute of Dental and Craniofacial Research (NIDCR).]

Sunil Wadhwa, Role of Estrogen Receptor Alpha and Beta in Regulating Mandibular Condylar Growth

Sunil Wadhwa is interested in the role estrogen receptors play in regulating mandibular condylar growth. Approximately 10 percent of the U.S. population has suffered from temporomandibular joint disorders (TMD). TMD predominantly affects women, but the reasons behind this are unknown. Dr. Wadhwa's research examines the mechanism behind estrogen inhibition of growth and differentiation of the mandibular condylar cartilage, which will give further insight into the age and gender predilection of TMD. His major research focus for the last five years has been on examining the molecular pathways that regulate temporomandibular joint mechanical loading–induced remodeling. [Funded by the National Institute of Dental and Craniofacial Research (NIDCR).]

NEUROSCIENCE AND PAIN

Jeremy Mao, Multidisciplinary Training in Temporomandibular Joint Disorders/Pain: Integrating Basic, Translational, and Clinical Science

Developing the research careers of junior faculty becomes an important pipeline for the future. Using the study of temporomandibular pain disorders as a theme, this K–12 training grant has three training tracks: genetics/physiology, bioengineering/regeneration, and imaging/biomechanics. A select group of young investigators who have shown the interest and ability to grow into independent researchers will have the opportunity to train in one of these tracks over the course of the five-year grant period. [Funded by the National Institute of Dental and Craniofacial Research (NIDCR).]

Kavita Ahluwalia, Research Supplement to Promote Diversity in Health-related Research, funded by the NIH/National Institute on Aging via Weill Medical College of Cornell University

Kavita Ahluwalia's research is aimed at improving the health and well-being of older adults who suffer from pain or who are at risk for pain. While a member of the Translational Research Institute on Pain in Later Life (TRIPLL), a multi-institutional, interdisciplinary collaborative team focused on the translation of basic behavioral and social science research into treatments that improve the well-being of older adults who suffer from pain, she contributed to the development of innovative methods and strategies that facilitate such treatment while focusing on the oral health of homebound elders.

MICROBIAL PATHOGENESIS/MICROBIOME

Yiping Han, *Fusobacterium nucleatum*–mediated Stimulation of Colorectal Cancer: Mechanistic Studies

Yiping Han, Investigation of FadA Adhesin from *Fusobacterium nucleatum* R01

Yiping Han is studying drivers of colorectal cancer (CRC), which is the second leading cause of cancer death in the United States. *Fusobacterium nucleatum*, a common oral bacterium, has recently been indicated to stimulate CRC. This study, funded by the NIH/National Cancer Institute, investigates how *F. nucleatum* drives CRC. The results will advance understanding of colorectal carcinogenesis and identify novel diagnostic and therapeutic targets for CRC. In further studies, Dr. Han and her team have discovered that *F. nucleatum* uniquely stimulates the growth of colorectal cancer cells, but not breast cancer cells or colorectal adenoma cells, suggesting such stimulation requires specific host somatic mutations. In this further research her team is investigating the host genomic determinants of such stimulation.

Yiping Han, Mechanism of *Fusobacterium nucleatum* in Intrauterine Infection

Yiping Han is also studying mechanisms of intrauterine infection, a major cause of pregnancy complications such as preterm birth and stillbirth. *Fusobacterium nucleatum*, a common oral bacterium, is one of the most prevalent species in intrauterine infection. Using a highly integrated and state-of-the-art approach, Dr. Han's laboratory analyzes the pathogenesis mechanisms of *F. nucleatum* in intrauterine infection to identify potential targets to treat and prevent intrauterine infection. Results from the study will impact understanding of this serious infectious disease and patient management. Moreover, they will shed novel light on how oral bacteria impact infections and inflammation at extra-oral sites. [Funded by the National Institute of Dental and Craniofacial Research (NIDCR).]

BEHAVIORAL SCIENCES/HEALTH SCIENCES

David Albert, Developing a Decision Support System to Promote Tobacco Counseling by Dentists

Over the past fifteen years David Albert has investigated ways to integrate tobacco cessation interventions into the health-care setting. His earlier work has led him to the development of a clinical decision support system (CDSS) to promote tobacco counseling by dentists. Input from general practitioners will inform the development and pilot testing of this innovative health-care information technology aimed at promoting the application of tobacco cessation guidelines in general practice dental offices. The study team will assemble an expert panel, convene focus groups, develop and design the CDSS, and pilot test the system to evaluate its adoption and maintenance. [Funded by the National Institute of Dental and Craniofacial Research (NIDCR).]

Burton Edelstein, Planning a Stage II Trial to Prevent ECC Progression

Burton Edelstein's planning grant aims to develop a behavioral randomized controlled trial (B-RCT) of the MySmileBuddy intervention to test the effectiveness of this innovative, family-centered, technology-assisted behavioral intervention to manage early childhood caries among affected low-income Hispanic children. If successful, the proposed intervention will reduce disease progression in a highly vulnerable population, promote a shift in current practice of pediatric dentistry toward disease prevention and control, and represent a significant step toward reducing ethnic-racial disparities in oral health. [Funded by the National Institute of Dental and Craniofacial Research (NIDCR).]

Carol Kunzel, Integrating Social and Systems Science Approaches to Promote Oral Health Equity

Carol Kunzel is studying the integration of social and systems science approaches to promote oral health equity. Demographic shifts that include an aging and more racially and ethnically diverse population coupled with ongoing changes in the health-care policy environment are demanding that the dental profession both redirect and expand its focus. Her research focuses on how factors at multiple scales contribute to oral health and care-seeking behaviors for racial and ethnic minority older adults. The results aim to enhance community and clinic-based oral health service delivery and improve oral health outcomes in this population. [Funded by the National Institute of Dental and Craniofacial Research (NIDCR).]

SYSTEMIC AND ORAL DISEASE INTERACTIONS

Evanthia Lalla, Secondary Analysis of EHR Data to Enhance Care of Dental Patients with Diabetes

Evanthia Lalla's research aims to (1) identify people with undiagnosed diabetes or at risk for diabetes and (2) determine the impact of certain diabetes parameters on oral health and on the response to (and recovery from) dental procedures. Because of the tremendous health and financial burden diabetes places on our nation, the work is highly relevant to the public's health. Using data from the Marshfield Clinic's electronic medical and dental record system, the research seeks to find the best model to identify existing undiagnosed diabetes and prediabetes among dental patients; to forecast incident disease over a five-year period among dental patients; and to determine the burden of diabetic patients' levels of glycemic control on their oral/periodontal disease status over time, their response to therapy, and their healing following oral/periodontal surgery and/or tooth extractions. [Funded by the National Institute of Dental and Craniofacial Research (NIDCR).]

Panos Papapanou, Genomic Approaches to the Pathobiology and Classification of Periodontitis, funded by the NIDCR

In this work, Panos Papapanou studies an available integrated database that includes demographic, clinical, microbiological, serological, genomic, and epigenetic data from 120 patients with moderate/severe periodontal disease in a systems biology approach to the study of the pathobiology and classification of human periodontitis.

Panos Papapanou, Periodontitis Exposure and Risk of Incident Dementia

Panos Papapanou's work addresses a growing body of evidence that supports an association between periodontitis and dementia, including Alzheimer's disease (AD) and related disorders. By examining oral health in a longitudinal manner within an established, rigorously developed, diverse community–based aging study in northern Manhattan (WHICAP), this study presents a unique opportunity to explore clinical and subclinical markers of periodontal disease in relation to markers of dementia, including neurological examination cognitive testing and disease indicators on multimodal neuroimaging and in blood. The study formally tests the hypothesis that periodontitis is an unrecognized risk factor for incident cognitive impairment among the participants in the WHICAP cohort currently being enrolled. [Funded by the National Institute of Dental and Craniofacial Research (NIDCR).]

Panos Papapanou, MicroRNA Expression in Gingival Tissues in Periodontal Health and Disease

Panos Papapanou is also studying the relevance of microRNAs in gingival tissues and their cellular components in periodontal health and disease. This study aims to validate the identified miRNAs' gene targets and examine their potential functions using in vitro studies. The data will ultimately contribute to a better understanding of the pathobiology of periodontal diseases. [Funded by the National Institute of Dental and Craniofacial Research (NIDCR).]

Ulrike Schulze-Späte, BRN3 Transcription Factor Family in Osteoclastogenesis

Ulrike Schulze-Späte's work revolves around bone resorption, a central mechanism in skeletal development, remodeling, and pathology. Resorption is mediated by osteoclasts, multinucleated giant cells that are derived from the monocyte/macrophage lineage. RANKL is a mandatory factor in inducing osteoclast differentiation, although the signaling pathways it activates are only partially understood. Previous work by Schulze-Späte identified the BRN3 transcription factor family as downstream targets of RANKL. The overall goal is to characterize BRN3 transcription factors and their target genes that are present in osteoclasts and determine their role in the regulation of bone under physiological and pathological conditions. [Funded by the National Institute of Dental and Craniofacial Research (NIDCR).]

Appendix 5

Members of the College of Dental Medicine Board of Advisors

In the 1980s a board of advisors was established to assist the dean in carrying out the school's missions. The role of the board is expanding to assist the College of Dental Medicine in making the shifts necessary for the future. The members of the board of advisors during the 2014–2015 year were as follows:

LESLIE W. SELDIN, DDS, 1966, Chair (an alumnus of the CDM)
CHARLES HAPCOOK, DDS, Eastern Dentists Insurance Company
JOEL HODGE, MBA, Aetna Dental, Inc.
DAVID JOSZA, MBA, Zimmer Biomet
KENNETH W. M. JUDY, DDS, International Congress of Oral Implantologists
STEVE KESS, BBA, MBA, Henry Schein, Inc.
MARC CRAWFORD LEAVITT, JD, Leavitt & Kerson, LLC
R. IVÁN LUGO, DMD, MBA, MSC, Procter & Gamble
MADELINE MONACO, PhD, MS, MEd, Johnson & Johnson Consumer and Personal Products Worldwide
FOTINOS S. PANAGAKOS, DMD, Colgate-Palmolive Company

ALUMNI/FACULTY MEMBERS

THOMAS J. CONNOLLY, DDS, 1977, Periodontics, 1980
JULIE A. CONNOLLY, DDS/MPH, 2001, Periodontics, 2005
ALEX DELL, DDS, 1959

Lois A. Jackson, DDS, 1977, Pediatric Dentistry, 1980
Margot H. Jaffe, DDS, 1980, Pediatric Dentistry, 1981, Orthodontics, 1985
Gabriela N. Lee, DDS, 1987
Michael Leifert, DDS, Orthodontics, 2004
James A. Lipton, DDS, 1971, PhD, Graduate School of Arts and Science 1980
Gregg S. Lituchy, DDS, 1984
Renee Litvak, DDS, 2002, Endodontics, 2004
Thomas J. Magnani, DDS, 1980
David Momtaheni, DMD (Faculty Member)

Appendix 6

Presidents of the Alumni Organization

The alumni organization has been an important link between the school and its graduates. The leadership of the organization is listed chronologically below:

1926–1930 Joseph Schroff

1930–1932 Joseph Horn

1936–1937 Manuel Maslansky

1937–1938 Frederick Birnberg

1938–1940 James Dunning

1940–1942 John Mayers

1942–1943 Philip Sueskind

1943–1944 Louis Citron

1944–1945 Donald Waugh

1945–1946 Louis Abelson

1946–1947 Edward White

1947–1948 Julius Horn

1948–1949 Morris Fierstein

1949–1950 William Giblin Jr.

1950–1951 Nathaniel Diner

1951–1952 John Flynn

1952–1953 Hannah Appel

1953–1954 Herman Malter

1954–1955 Joel Friedman

1955–1956 Lester Eisner

1956–1957 Bernard Sussman

1957–1958 Alex Lifschutz

1958–1959 Arthur Kulick

1959–1960 Robin Rankow

1960–1961 Samuel Rosenthal

1961 Jacob Friedlander

1961–1962 Fred Birnberg

1962–1963 George Kudler

1963–1964 Harold Cobin

1964–1965 Bert Schdeneman

1966–1967 Herman Ivahoe

1967–1968 Nathan Sheckman

1968–1969 George O'Grady

1969–1970 Lillian Bachman

1970–1971 Gerald Leberman

1971–1972 Matthew Levin

1972–1974 Frances Karlan

1974–1976 Morton Shapiro

1976–1978 William Jacobs

1978–1980 Edgar Gattegno

1980–1982 Sidney Shapiro

1982–1984 Richard Lichtenthal

1984–1986 Charles Solomon

1986–1988 Albert Thompson

1988–1990 Daniel Epstein

1990–1992 Olga Ibsen

1992–1994 Stuart Epstein

1994–1996 Jack Roth

1996–1998 James Abjanich

1998–2000 Daniel Zedeker

2000–2002 Joseph Ciccio

2002–2004 David Pitman

2004–2006 Sarina Reddy

2006–2008 Lois Jackson

2008–2011 Margot Jaffe

2011–2013 Renee Litvak

2013–2015 Julie Connolly

Appendix 7

Columbia University Alumni Distinguished Service Medal Awardees

This medal is awarded for distinguished service of ten years or more to the University, including its schools, alumni associations, regional Columbia clubs, and University-wide initiatives. The Alumni Medal was first awarded in 1933. Below are the recipients of the medal from the School of Dental and Oral Surgery.

1933: Joseph Horn, 1926

1945: James Dunning, 1930

1949: John Mayers, 1932

1954: Herman Malter, 1927

1959: Joel Friedman, 1939

1961: Arthur Kulick, 1926

1962: Alexander Lifschutz, 1926

1964: Samuel Rosenthal, 1925

1968: Harold Cobin, 1931

1971: Nathan Sheckman, 1938

1972: Morris Fierstein, 1921

1973: Matthew Levin, 1926

1974: Herman Ivahoe, 1931

1976: Nathaniel Diner, 1938

1977: Morton Shapiro, 1950

1979: William Jacobs, 1945

1980: Frances Karlan, 1949

1981: Edgar Gattegno, 1945

1982: Sidney Shapiro, 1948

1983: Richard Lichtenthal, 1962

1986: Charles Solomon, 1955

1988: Albert Thompson, 1960

1990: Daniel Epstein, 1953

1993: Olga Ibsen, 1972, 1975 (Dental Hygiene)

1997: Stuart Epstein, 1974

1999: Jack Roth, 1981

2000: Mark Tenner, 1962

2001: James Abjanich, 1983

2004: Daniel Zedeker, 1983

2006: Joseph Ciccio, 1983

2007: Alexandra Baranetsky, 1980

2009: Lois Jackson, 1977, Pediatric Dentistry 1980

2011: Margot Jaffe, 1981, Pediatric Dentistry 1981, Orthodontics 1985

2013: Leslie Seldin, 1966

2015: Thomas Connolly, 1977, Periodontics 1980

Appendix 8

College of Dental Medicine Distinguished Alumni Awardees

Beginning in 1990, the School of Dental and Oral Surgery/College of Dental Medicine began to recognize its graduates with notable accomplishments with a Distinguished Alumni Award. Listed below are those so awarded through 2014.

1990: Timothy Turvey (SDOS 1971) for achievement in the field of oral and maxillofacial surgery and at the University of North Carolina

1991: James Dunning (SDOS 1930) for achievement in academia as dean of the Harvard School of Dental Medicine

1991: Leslie Seldin (SDOS 1966) for service to the profession as president of the New York Dental Society and first vice president of the American Dental Association

1992: Paula Friedman (SDOS 1974) for service as president of the American Association of Dental Schools (now known as the American Dental Education Association)

1994: Caswell Evans (SDOS 1970) for achievement in the field of public health and as project director and executive editor of the landmark *Oral Health in America: A Report of the Surgeon General* (2000)

1995: Elizabeth (Bessie) Delany (SDOS 1923) for service to the Harlem community and for telling her story in the best-selling book *Having Our Say*

1996: Mark Tenner (SDOS 1962) for longtime volunteer faculty service to the College of Dental Medicine

1997: Lawrence Tabak (SDOS 1977) for achievement in research and as director of the National Institute of Dental and Craniofacial Research and principal deputy director of the National Institutes of Health

1998: Albert Thompson (SDOS 1960) for service to the University sports program and to the School of Dental and Oral Surgery in minority affairs

1999: Arthur Bushel (SDOS 1943, and School of Public Health 1947) for achievement in the field of public health dentistry and for work in adding fluoride to New York City's water supply

2000: Charles Solomon (SDOS 1958) for service to the College of Dental Medicine

2002: Paul Baer (SDOS 1945, and Periodontics 1955) for achievement in academia in the field of periodontology

2003: Samuel Pritz (SDOS 1933) for service to School of Dental and Oral Surgery/College of Dental Medicine as a member of the admission committee and adviser to the administration

2004: Ronald Dubner (SDOS 1958) for achievement in the field of the neuroscience of pain

2005: Syngcuk Kim (SDOS 1976, Endodontics 1978, and PhD, Graduate School of Arts and Sciences 1981) for achievement in academia in the field of dental pulp physiology

2006: Margot Jaffe (SDOS 1980, Pediatric Dentistry 1981, and Orthodontics 1985) for service to the College of Dental Medicine as alumni organization president and as a longtime volunteer faculty member

2007: Ralph Kaslick (SDOS 1959 and Periodontics 1972) for achievement in academia as dean of the Fairleigh Dickinson School of Dentistry and provost of the University

2008: John Scarola (SDOS 1960) for achievement in dental organization as president of the American College of Dentists and service to the school as a longtime volunteer faculty member

2009: Steven Syrop (SDOS 1980) for service to the College of Dental Medicine and for leadership in the field of temporomandibular disorders

2010: Louis Mandel (SDOS 1946) for service to the College of Dental Medicine and for achievement in research on the diseases of the salivary glands

2011: Brian Alpert (SDOS 1967) for achievement in academia in the field of oral and maxillofacial surgery at the University of Louisville, College of Dentistry

2012: Louis Rubins (SDOS 1960) for service to the College of Dental Medicine of more than forty years as a volunteer faculty member

2013: Martin Davis (SDOS 1974 and Pediatric Dentistry 1975) for service to the College of Dental Medicine as director of the Division of Pediatric Dentistry, head of the Section of Comprehensive Care, and associate dean for student and alumni affairs, and for achievement as president of the American Association of Pediatric Dentistry and president of the American Society of Dentistry for Children

2014: Thomas Magnani (SDOS 1980) for service to the College of Dental Medicine as president of the 1852 Society

Appendix 9

A Snapshot of Distinguished Graduates
of the College of Dental Medicine

Many graduates have distinguished themselves in organized dentistry, in academia, and in research. Listed here are some outstanding examples.

Columbia graduates Percy Phillips (DDS 1919) and Louis Saporito (DDS 1922) have led the American Dental Association (ADA); Dr. Phillips became the president of the Dental Society of the State of New York and the president of the ADA. Dr. Leslie Seldin (SDOS 1966), was vice president of the ADA and president of the New York State Dental Society. Seldin now serves as chair of the College of Dental Medicine Advisory Council. And recently, Jonathan Shenkin (SDOS 1996) served as vice president of the ADA and president of the Maine Dental Association. Shenkin also was selected as a Fulbright Scholar in 2015.

Other graduates such as Dr. John Scarola (DDS 1960) served as president of the American College of Dentists; Dr. Robert Gottsegen (DDS 1943 and Periodontics 1948) served as president of the American Academy of Periodontology; Dr. John Lucca (DDS 1948) served as president of the Greater New York Academy of Prosthodontists; Martin Davis (DDS 1974 and Pediatric Dentistry 1975) served as president of the American Association of Pediatric Dentistry and president of the American Society of Pediatric Dentistry; Dr. George Lacovara (SDOS 1962) served as president of the Connecticut State Dental Association.

And two Columbians became presidents of organizations that William Gies founded: Irwin Mandel (SDOS 1945) served as president of the American Association of Dental Research, founded in 1919. And in 2003 Paula Friedman (SDOS 1974) served as president of the American Association of Dental Schools (now called the American Dental Education Association), founded in 1923.

Still other examples of graduates who have distinguished themselves as deans of dental schools, chairs of departments, and in government service are: James Dunning (SDOS 1941) served as dean of the Harvard School of Dental Medicine; Maurice Hickey (DMD, Harvard 1932, and MD Columbia Physicians and Surgeons 1937) served as associate dean of SDOS and then dean at the University of Washington; Dr. Ralph Kaslick (SDOS 1959 and Periodontics 1962) served as dean of the Fairleigh Dickinson College of Dental Medicine; Robert Saporito (SDOS 1961) served as dean of the New Jersey Dental School and vice president for academic affairs at the University of Medicine and Dentistry of New Jersey; Dr. Allan Kucine (SDOS 1982) served as associate dean for Information Technology, State University of New York, Stony Brook, School of Dental Medicine; Dr. Syngcuk Kim (SDOS 1976, and PhD, Graduate School of Arts and Sciences 1978) serves as chair of the Department of Endodontics, University of Pennsylvania School of Dentistry; Dana Graves (SDOS 1980) served as chairman of the Department of Periodontics at the New Jersey Dental School and, subsequently, chair of the Department of Periodontics at the University of Pennsylvania School of Dentistry; Dr. Joan Phelan (BS, Columbia Dental Hygiene 1962, MS 1967, and DMD, SUNY Stony Brook) serves as chair of the Department of Oral Pathology at the New York University College of Dentistry. Dr. Jessica Lee (SDOS 1997) is currently serving as chair of the Department of Pediatric Dentistry at the University of North Carolina Chapel Hill School of Dental Medicine.

Dr. Lawrence Tabak (SDOS 1977) is distinguished for his service as director of the National Institute of Dental and Craniofacial Research from 2000 to 2008 and, subsequently, his appointment as principal deputy director of the National Institutes of Health in 2010, a position he currently holds. Dr. Caswell Evans (SDOS 1970) served as director of public health programs and services for the Los Angeles County Department of Public Health, president of the American Public Health Association and the American Association of Public Health Dentistry, and as the executive editor and project manager for *Oral Health in America: A*

Report of the Surgeon General (2000). He currently serves as associate dean for prevention and public health at the College of Dentistry at the University of Illinois at Chicago. Dr. Renee Joskow (SDOS 1985 and MPH School of Public Health 1985) serves as the senior advisor for oral health and chief dental officer of the Health Resources and Services Administration of the U.S. Department of Health and Human Services. She previously served as senior medical epidemiologist for the U.S. Department of Homeland Security.

Appendix 10

The Deans of the Dental School and Directors of the Dental Hygiene Program

The leadership of the dental school had various titles over the past 100 years reflecting the organizational setup. At its inception, the school was administered under the Columbia University Extension Center, with the director of the Extension Center responsible for the school. Between 1933 and 1958, the dean of the medical school also served as dean of the dental school, with associate deans responsible for day-to-day operations. After the School of Dental Hygiene was incorporated into the dental school in 1917, the school became a program of the dental school led by a director.

1916–1920 James Chidester Egbert, PhD, director of the University Extension Center
1920–1927 Frank Thorn Van Woert, Master of Dental Science
1927–1933 Alfred Owre, DMD, MD, dean
1933–1958 Willard Rappleye, MD, dean of SDOS and P&S

ASSOCIATE DEANS IN CHARGE OF OPERATION OF THE SDOS UNDER THE ADMINISTRATION OF DEAN RAPPLEYE

1933–1935 Arthur Rowe, DDS
1935–1945 Houghton Holiday, DDS
1946–1949 Bion East, DDS
1949–1956 Maurice Hickey, DMD, MD
1956–1958 Gilbert Smith, DDS

DEANS

1959–1968 Gilbert Smith, DDS
1968–1973 Melvin Moss, DDS, PhD
1973–1978 Edward Zegarelli, DDS
1978–2001 Allan Formicola, DDS, MS
2001–2011 Ira Lamster, DMD, MMSc
2011–2013 Ronnie Myers, DDS, (interim)
2013–present Christian Stohler, DMD, DrMedDent

DENTAL HYGIENE DIRECTORS

1917–1920 Louise C. Ball, DDS
1920–1947 Anna Hughes, DMD
1947–1965 Frances A. Stoll, RDH, MA
1965–1977 Patricia McLean, RDH, MA
1977–1988 Dona Wayman, BS, MS, EdD

Appendix 11

Milestones in the History of the College of Dental Medicine: 1916–2016

What follows is a list of events or milestones, which had major impact on the College of Dental Medicine since its establishment in 1916.

1916: Founding Document "A Dental School on University Lines" is completed by the Committee for Columbia University Dental School consisting of members from the College of Physicians and Surgeons and leading dentists in New York.

1917: Columbia University Trustees approve the establishment of the dental school retroactively to September 17, 1916. Two students enroll.

1917: The New York Post-graduate School of Dentistry and the New York School of Dental Hygiene are merged into the Columbia University Dental School.

1919: The Columbia University Dental School is the first school in the nation to require two years of prerequisite college preparation as an entry requirement.

1919: William J. Gies forms the *Journal of Dental Research.*

1920: A building for the dental school is constructed next to the College of Physicians and Surgeons building on West Fifty-Ninth Street.

1923: The College of Dental and Oral Surgery, which dates back to a New York State charter in 1852, is absorbed by the Columbia University Dental School. The two buildings the College occupied on East Thirty-Fourth and Thirty-Fifth Street become Columbia University property. The Columbia University Dental School changes its name to the School of Dental and Oral Surgery.

1926: The Carnegie Foundation for the Advancement of Teaching publishes *Dental Education in the United Sates and Canada*, prepared by William J. Gies, one of the key founders of the dental school and guiding light for its inception.

1928: The School of Dental and Oral Surgery moves to three floors in the newly constructed Columbia–Presbyterian Medical Center Vanderbilt Clinic building next to the College of Physicians and Surgeons building.

1933: The dean of the medical school also becomes the dean of the dental school and appoints associate deans to carry out day-to-day operations.

1935: Associate dean Arthur Rowe and faculty member Paul Wiberg are murdered by Victor Koussow, a deranged school laboratory technician.

1945: Formal merger of the dental school into the Faculty of Medicine. The school becomes the SDOS of the Faculty of Medicine.

1947: The Council on Dental Education of the American Dental Association, the accrediting body for dental schools, drops SDOS from accredited schools due to its merger under the Faculty of Medicine.

1951: The Council on Dental Education restores SDOS to the list of approved schools.

1959: The SDOS separates from the Faculty of Medicine. The University approves a separate faculty, the Faculty of Dental and Oral Surgery. The associate dean's position under the former arrangement is restored to dean.

1963: SDOS placed on provisional accreditation by the Council of Dental Education due to facility and equipment issues and inadequate representation of the school within the Medical Center.

1972: SDOS regains full accreditation after improving facilities, a status it maintains throughout the next three decades.

1976: SDOS is awarded New York State funding and becomes a private, state-related school, reserving 70 percent of its seats for New York State residents.

1977: SDOS facilities on Vanderbilt Clinic floors 7, 8, and 9 and completes a total renovation and update with modern equipment.

1982: The MD oral and maxillofacial surgery residency program is established between SDOS, P&S, and the Presbyterian Hospital. It is the seventh such program in the nation.

1983: A master of arts degree program for postdoctoral students is established through the Graduate School of Arts and Sciences.

1986: SDOS is selected to receive funding from the Pew Foundation to implement far-reaching strategic changes in its curriculum and patient care programs. Joint degree opportunities are made available for students through an area of concentration program for degrees in public health and business.

1988: New York State stops providing capitation support for the private medical and dental schools in the state and reduces the clinic support for SDOS. SDOS becomes a private school again. The DDS student body shifts from one predominantly from New York State to one representative of many states and countries.

1988: The Harlem Hospital-SDOS special postdoctoral residency program is established to educate underrepresented minority residents in the dental specialties.

1992: SDOS gains expansion spaces on Presbyterian Hospital's seventh floor (East, Center and Stem) in the building at 168th Street.

1993: SDOS establishes the Columbia Dental Plan to provide dental care to university faculty.

1995: SDOS reaches out into the community and establishes the Community Dent-Care Network to provide care in public schools and Head Start centers.

2005: SDOS begins a global outreach initiative to promote collaborations with international dental schools.

2006: The board of trustees approves a name change to the College of Dental Medicine to reflect its comprehensive biomedical approach in its missions.

2008: New academic space is made available on the seventeenth floor of the Presbyterian Hospital building.

2009: The College of Dental Medicine receives the American Dental Education Association William J. Gies Foundation Award for Outstanding Vision by an Academic Dental Institution.

2009: A major new research complex is constructed on the twelfth floor of the Vanderbilt Clinic building.

2010: A DDS-MA program with Teachers College is established.

2014: CDM wins a second American Dental Education Association William J. Gies Foundation Award for Outstanding Achievement by an Academic Dental Institution for its Community DentCare program.

2014: CDM is awarded a Higher Education Excellence to Diversity Award for outstanding commitment to diversity and inclusion, the first dental school in the nation to win such an award.

2015: CDM acquires the fifth floor of the Vanderbilt Clinic for expansion space.

2016: CDM celebrates its 100th anniversary.

Notes

1. 1916–1941: A DENTAL SCHOOL ON UNIVERSITY LINES

1. "The Unlicensed Dentists," *New York Times*, September 26, 1909, http://timesmachine .nytimes.com/timesmachine/1909/09/26/110035799.html?pageNumber=12.
2. "Crusading Against the City's Unethical Dentists: The Day of the Bargain Dental Parlor Where Patients Were Maltreated and Fleeced Is Passing," *New York Times*, September 18, 1910, http://timesmachine.nytimes.com/timesmachine /1910/09/18/issue.html.
3. *A Dental School on University Lines* (New York: Columbia University, May 1916).
4. The name of the College of Dental Medicine changed over the years: it was the Columbia University Dental School in the founding document (1916–1923); this was changed to the School of Dental and Oral Surgery in 1923 on the merger with the College of Dental and Oral Surgery (1923–2006); and it was renamed the College of Dental Medicine in 2006 to reflect the current mission of the College.
5. William J. Gies, "Mouth Bacteria: An Essay Presented to the Canadian Oral Prophylactic Association." *Journal of the American College of Dentists* 79, no. 2 (2012): 5–11.
6. William J. Gies, "Dental Education in the United States and Canada: A Report to the Carnegie Foundation for the Advancement of Teaching," *Bulletin* 19 (1926): 191.
7. Frank J. Orland, *William John Gies: His Contributions to the Advancement of Dentistry* (Alexandria, Va.: William J. Gies Foundation with special assistance of the International Association for Dental Research, 1992).

8. Netta Wilson, *Alfred Owre: Dentistry's Militant Educator* (Minneapolis: University of Minnesota Press, 1937), 22.

9. Central files, box 352 (folder 6), Alfred Owre, Archives and Special Collections, Butler Library, Columbia University.

10. Wilson, *Alfred Owre*, 111–112.

11. David Nash. "Alfred Owre: Revisiting the Thought of a Distinguished, Though Controversial Early Twentieth-Century Dental Educator," *Journal of Dental Education* 77, no. 8 (2013): 972–981.

12. *Columbia Dentor*, vol. 1 (New York: published by the student body of the School of Dental and Oral Surgery of Columbia University, 1928), Foreword.

13. Frank Thorn Van Woert, letter of January 18, 1926, to Henry Gillett, SDOS Historical Collection 1892–1989, box 1, Archives and Special Collections. Augustus C. Long Health Sciences Library, Columbia University Medical Center.

14. Columbia University in the City of New York, announcement of the School of Dental and Oral Surgery, 1933–1934, page 22 of the bulletin.

15. Edward Kovar, *Columbia Daily Spectator*, December 13, 1935. http://spectator archive.library.columbia.edu/cgi-bin/columbia?a=d&d=cs19351213-01.1.1&e= ------en-20--1--txt-txIN-----.

16. Nathan Sheckman, telephone interview conducted by Allan J. Formicola, June 1, 2015. Sheckman was 102 years old at the time. He was well and living in an assisted-living senior citizens' center in Fort Myers, Fla.

17. "Clinic Slayer Sane, Doctors Ruled in '27," *New York Post*, December 13, 1935.

18. Houghton Holiday, statement in the *Dental Columbian*, 1937.

19. Alfred Owre, "Report of the Dean of the Dental School" (1929).

20. Personal communication with Martin J. Davis, formerly director of pedodontics, associate dean for student and alumni affairs at Columbia University, College of Dental Medicine, and past president of the American Academy of Pediatric Dentistry.

2. 1941–1978: LIVING UP TO STANDARDS: THE DIFFICULT YEARS

1. Statement by President Butler concerning new plan of dental education and research in Columbia University, Vice President's Central Records, box 308, General Correspondence of the School of Dentistry, Archives and Special Collections, Augustus C. Long Health Sciences Library, Columbia University Medical Center.

2. Dean's Annual Report, 1933. Note: Rappleye prepared the dean's annual report to the University after the leave of Owre and for the remainder of the merger period. Available in the Annual Report of the President and Treasurer to the

Trustees, June 30, 1933, page 306. Accessed April 23, 2016 at https://archive.org/details/annualreport1933colu.

3. The American Dental Association's Council on Dental Education was the predecessor of the Commission on Dental Accreditation.

4. These included Nicholas DiSalvo (DDS, SDOS 1945), who completed a PhD in physiology in 1952; Melvin Moss (DDS, SDOS 1946), who earned the PhD in anatomy in 1954; Solon (Art) Ellison (DDS, SDOS 1946), Moss's classmate, who earned the PhD in microbiology in 1958; Herbert Bartelstone (DDS, SDOS 1945), who earned the PhD in pharmacology in 1960; and Norman Kahn (DDS, SDOS 1958), who was awarded the PhD in pharmacology in 1964. Each of these individuals was appointed in the respective basic science departments of physiology, anatomy, microbiology, and pharmacology.

5. Columbia University, press release, February 23, 1957, Vice President's Central Records, box 308, Central Files, General Correspondence Dental School 1951–1975, Archives and Special Collections, Augustus C. Long Health Sciences Library, Columbia University Medical Center.

6. Report of the Trustees' Ad Hoc Committee on the School of Dental and Oral Surgery, box 308, Central Files, General Correspondence Dental School 1951–1975, Archives and Special Collections, Augustus C. Long Health Sciences Library, Columbia University Medical Center.

7. Dr. Letty Moss-Salentijn, personal conversation with Allan J. Formicola, June 30, 2015.

3. 1978–2001: THE LEAP TO THE FUTURE

1. ADA, Report of the Special Higher Education Committee to Critique the 1976 Dental Curriculum Study. Issues in Dental Health Policy.

2. Author's note: I wrote this chapter in the third person rather than in the first person, although it covers the twenty-three years of my deanship. I followed the same protocol in researching this chapter for this period of time as I did for the previous chapters, that is, I took the information from the archives in the Long Library. The library collected the papers from my deanship. As I researched the information, it seemed more appropriate to write the chapter in the third person in order for me to stay objective rather than to make this a personal account of the time I served as dean.

3. Irwin Mandel obituary and guestbook, *New York Times*, May 28, 2011, accessed July 26, 2015, www.legacy.com/guestbooks/nytimes/Irwin-d-mandel-condolences/151330661?&page=2.

4. Allan J. Formicola, S. Marshall, and N. Kahn, "Strengthening the Education of the General Dentist for the 21st Century," *Journal of Dental Education* 54, no. 2 (1990): 109–114.

5. V. Evangelidis-Sakellson, "Student Productivity Under Requirement and Comprehensive Care Systems," *Journal of Dental Education* 63, no. 5 (1999): 407–413.

6. Allan J. Formicola, "The Dental Curriculum: The Interplay of Pragmatic Necessities, National Needs, and Educational Philosophies in Shaping Its Future," *Journal of Dental Education* 55, no. 6 (1991): 358–364.

7. S. Marshall, A. Formicola, and J. McIntosh, "Columbia University's Community Dental Programs as Framework for Education," *Journal of Dental Education* 63, no. 12 (1999): 944–946.

8. Allan J. Formicola and Lourdes Hernandez-Cordero, *Mobilizing the Community for Better Health: What the Rest of America Can Learn from Northern Manhattan*, New York: Columbia University Press, 2010.

9. Felicia R. Lee, "Polishing Columbia's Bad-Neighbor Image." *New York Times*, September 9, 2001.

4. 2001–2013: THE NEW MILLENNIUM

1. Author's note: This chapter was drafted by Ira Lamster, DMD, MMSc, and dean emeritus. Dr. Ronnie Myers, DDS, drafted the section on the interim deanship.

2. Records of the Office of the Dean (College of Dental Medicine/Lamster), Archives & Special Collections, Augustus C. Long Health Sciences Library, Columbia University Medical Center; Boxes 1–3.

3. Ira Lamster, "Oral Health Care Services for Older Adults: A Looming Crisis," *American Journal of Public Health* 94, no. 5 (May 2004): 699–702.

4. S. Marshall, M. E. Northridge, L. D. De La Cruz, R. D. Vaughan, J. O'Neil-Dunne, and I. B. Lamster, "ElderSmile: A Comprehensive Approach to Improving Oral Health for Seniors," *American Journal of Public Health* 99, no. 4 (April 2009): 595–599.

5. Ira B. Lamster and Mary Northridge, eds., *Improving Oral Health for the Elderly: An Interdisciplinary Approach* (New York: Springer, 2008).

6. J. J. Mao, S. G. Kim, J. Zhou, L. Ye, S. Cho, T. Suzuki, S. Y. Fu, R. Yang, and X. Zhou, "Regenerative Endodontics: Barriers and Strategies for Clinical Translation," *Dental Clinics of North America* 56, no. 3 (July 2012): 639–649.

7. R. Graham, L. A. Zubiaurre Bitzer, O. R. Anderson, M. Klyvert, L. Moss-Salentijn, and I. B. Lamster, "Advancing the Educational Training of Dental Educators: Review of a Model Program," *Journal of Dental Education* 76, no. 3 (March 2012): 303–310.

8. L. Tabak and S. Turner. "The Importance of Scientific Research and Teaching Critical Thinking in Academic Dental Institutions: Reactions to Dominic P. DePaola's 'The Revitalization of U.S. Dental Education,'" supplement, *Journal of Dental Education* 72, no. 2 (2008): 43–45.

5. 2013–2016 AND BEYOND: PLANS FOR THE NEXT 100 YEARS

1. Mark Kac, "Synoptic Description of Talk Entitled 'Whither Stochastic Processes?'" *SIAM Review* 15, no. 1 (January 1973): 256.
2. Dr. Letty Moss-Salentijn, vice dean for academic affairs, presented this description of the curriculum. Dr. Louis Mandel, associate dean for extramural hospital programs provided the information for the hospital rotations.
3. Houghton Holiday, statement in the *Dental Columbian*, 1937.

6. STUDENTS AND ALUMNI

1. Allan J. Formicola, "Women: A Resource for Dental Education," 1993 *New York State Dental Journal* 59: 39–43.
2. S. Delany and A. E. Delany, with A. Hill Hearth, *Having Our Say: The Delany Sisters' First 100 Years* (New York: Dell/Random House, 1997).
3. *Journal of the William Jarvie Society* 56 (Spring 2013): 16.
4. "Primus notable: Ronald Dubner DDS '58, PHD '64," *Primus* (Fall 2005): inside back cover.
5. "*Primus* Notable: Paul N. Baer '45, Perio '55," *Primus* (Summer 2010): back cover.
6. "*Primus* Notable: Dana Graves '80," *Primus* (Summer 2009): back cover.
7. The students who attended the focus group were: Katie Cass and Al Huynh, class of 2018; Victor Lee and Alina O'Brien, class of 2017; Ralph Liy and Derek Chenet, class of 2016; Joseph Wang and Keith Goldman, second-year postdoctoral students in orthodontics and periodontics, respectively.

Bibliography

CHAPTER 1. 1916–1941: A DENTAL SCHOOL ON UNIVERSITY LINES

A Dental School on University Lines. New York: Columbia University, May 1916.

A Medical Center for New York: The Alliance Between Columbia University and Presbyterian Hospital. New York: Columbia University, May 1915.

Abraham Flexner. *Medical Education in the United States and Canada.* A Report to the Carnegie Foundation for the Advancement of Teaching. Bulletin Number Four. pub: D. B. Updike, Boston: Merrymount Press, 1910.

Archives and Special Collections. A. C. Long Health Sciences Library. Columbia University Medical Center. Statement by President Butler Concerning New Plan of Dental Education and Research in Columbia University. Box 308: General Correspondence of the School of Dentistry.

Archives and Special Collections. Butler Library. Columbia University. January 4, 1932, letter from Alfred Owre to Nicholas Murray Butler.

"Clinic Slayer Sane, Doctors ruled in '27." *New York Post,* December 13, 1935.

Columbia Dentor. Volume 1. New York: published by the student body of the School of Dental and Oral Surgery of Columbia University, 1928.

Columbia University in the City of New York. School of Dentistry Announcement 1917–1918 and through 1941. https://archive.org/details/announcement1917colu and https://archive.org/details/announcement1934colu.

"Crusading Against the City's Unethical Dentists: The Day of the Bargain Dental Parlor Where Patients Were Maltreated and Fleeced Is Passing." *New York Times,*

September 18, 1910. http://timesmachine.nytimes.com/timesmachine/1910/09/18
/issue.html.

Gies, W. J. "Additions to the Discussion of Professional Journalism Versus Supply-House
Journalism in Dentistry." *Journal of the Allied Dental Societies* 12, no. 3 (September
1917): 303–326.

——. "Another Illustration of the Need for Caution in the Interpretation of 'Results'
Obtained in Experiments." *Journal of the Allied Dental Societies* 12, no. 1 (March
1917): 59–64.

——. "Chemical Studies of the Relations of Oral Microorganisms to Dental Caries."
Journal of the Allied Dental Societies 12, no. 4 (December 1917): 463–470.

——. William J. Gies. "Dental Education in the United States and Canada: A Report
to the Carnegie Foundation for the Advancement of Teaching." *Bulletin* 19; pub.
D. B. Updike: Merrymount Press, Boston. 1926.

——. "Further Remarks on the Validity of Marshall's 'Salivary Factor' for the Bio-
chemical Determination of Susceptibility to, or Immunity from, Dental Caries."
Journal of the Allied Dental Societies 11, no. 3 (1916): 488–516.

——. "Independent Journalism Versus Trade Journalism in Dentistry." *Journal of the
Allied Dental Societies* 11, no. 4 (December 1916): 577–623.

——. "An Interesting Fact Regarding the Reaction of Saliva to Phenothalein." *Journal
of the Allied Dental Societies* 11, no. 2 (June 1916): 273–274.

——. "Mouth Bacteria: An Essay Presented to the Canadian Oral Prophylactic
Association." *Journal of the American College of Dentists* 79, no. 2 (2012):
5–11.

——. "New Findings in Studies of the Validity of Marshall's 'Salivary Factor' as a
Means of Diagnosis of Dental Caries." *Journal of the Allied Dental Societies* 12,
no. 2 (June 1917): 212–218.

——. "Supplementary Comment on the Validity of Marshall's 'Salivary Factors.'"
Journal of the Allied Dental Societies 11, no. 4 (December 1916): 659–667.

——. "New Findings in Studies of the Validity of Marshall's 'Salivary Factor' as a
Means of Diagnosis of Dental Caries." *Journal of the Allied Dental Societies* 12,
no. 2 (June 1917): 212–218.

Holiday, Houghton *Dental Columbian*, 1937.

Kovar, Edward. *Columbia Daily Spectator*. December 13, 1935, http://spectator
archive.library.columbia.edu/cgi-bin/columbia?a=d&d=cs19351213-01.1.1&e
=------en-20--1--txt-txIN-----.

Nash, D. "Alfred Owre: Revisiting the Thought of a Distinguished, Though Controversial Early Twentieth-Century Dental Educator." *Journal of Dental Education*
77, no. 8 (2013): 972–981.

Kurtz, M. "Columbia University and Those Who Made It the Mecca of Dental Education." *Bulletin of the History of Dentistry* 26, no. 2 (1978): 86–103.

Maslansky, Manuel. "Amos Westcott—And His Influence on Dental Education." *Journal of the Dental Society of the State of New York* March–April, 1940: 2–18.

Orland, Frank J. *William John Gies: His Contribution to the Advancement of Dentistry.* Alexandria, Va.: William J. Gies Foundation for the Advancement of Dentistry with special assistance from the International Association of Dental Research, 1992.

Owre, Alfred. "Report of the Dean of the Dental School." 1929. Augustus C. Long Library, Archives and Special Collections. School of Dental and Oral Surgery. Deans Annual Reports 1928–1945. Box 1, Columbia University Medical Center, NY.

"The Unlicensed Dentists." *New York Times,* Sept. 26, 1909. http://timesmachine .nytimes.com/timesmachine/1909/09/26/110035799. html?pageNumber=12.

Wilson, Netta W. *Alfred Owre: Dentistry's Militant Educator.* Minneapolis: University of Minnesota Press, 1937.

January 4, 1932, letter from Alfred Owre to Nicholas Murray Butler: Owre statement on dental schools to be incorporated into medical schools.

CHAPTER 2. 1941–1978: LIVING UP TO STANDARDS

Archives and Special Collections. Augustus C. Long Health Sciences Library. Columbia University Medical Center. Statement by President Butler Concerning New Plan of Dental Education and Research in Columbia University. Vice President's Central Records, Box 308: General Correspondence of the School of Dentistry.

- 1972 Accreditation Report from the Council of Dental Education
- Columbia University News Letter. "Alumni Honor Retiring Dean" 1973
- Letter from the Council on Dental Education to Dean Edward Zegarelli regarding progress report on recommendations
- Spectator "State Aid for Dental School Weighed," April 4, 1975
- September 11, 1975 letter to Dean Donald Tapley (P&S) from Dean Edward Zegarelli informing of the approval of the grant to renovate VC 7, 8, and 9 and the increase of class size from 52 to 60

Dean's Annual Report 1933. Augustus C. Long Library. Archives and Special Collections. SDOS Deans Annual reports 1928–1945. Box 1. Columbia University Medical Center, NY.

Dean's Annual Report, December 31, 1975: Combined Annual Report, Columbia University and the Presbyterian Hospital. Augustus C. Long Library. Archives and Special Collections, Columbia University Medical Center, NY.

CHAPTER 3. 1978–2001: THE LEAP TO THE FUTURE

Archives and Special Collections. Augustus C. Long Health Sciences Library. Columbia University Medical Center. Central Files Box 310: General Correspondence Dental School 1983–1995, available Archives and Special Collections, A.C. Long Health Sciences Library, Columbia University Medical Center

- Accreditation Review, 1979
- Advisory Committee for the SDOS Strategic Planning Project, 1987
- Committee to Recommend a Dental Plan for Faculty and Officers of the University, 1980
- Clinical Research Center for Dentistry, 1985

Central Files Boxes 312, 313, and 314: General Correspondence Dental School, available Archives and Special Collections, A.C. Long Health Sciences Library, Columbia University Medical Center

- Letter from Allan J. Formicola to John Westcott for a financial distress grant, November 14, 1978
- Health Sciences Loan to the SDOS (Dr. A. Formicola), 1992
- Implementation of Strategic Plan–Pew Memorial Trust (Dr. Formicola), 1987–1988
- Minutes of the Faculty, February 5, 1988
- Minutes of the Faculty, May 12, 1989
- Deans Report: 10 Year Summary 1978–1988 and major goals for 1989–1994

Evangelidis-Sakellson, V. "Student Productivity Under Requirement and Comprehensive Care Systems." *Journal of Dental Education* 63, no. 5 (1991): 407–413.

Formicola, A., "The Dental Curriculum: The Interplay of Pragmatic Necessities, National Needs, and Educational Philosophies in Shaping Its Future." *Journal of Dental Education* 55, no. 6 (1991): 358–364.

Formicola, A., and N. Kahn. "Basic Sciences Instruction, The Columbia University Model." *Journal of Dental Education* 56, no. 5 (1992): 341–345.

Formicola, A., S. Marshall, and N. Kahn. "Strengthening the Education of the General Dentist for the 21st Century." *Journal of Dental Education* 54, no. 2 (1990): 109–114.

Lee, Felicia R. "Polishing Columbia's Bad-Neighbor Image." *New York Times*, September 9, 2001.

Marshall, S., A. Formicola, and J. McIntosh. "Columbia University's Community Dental Program as a Framework for Education." *Journal of Dental Education*; 63, no. 12 (1999): 944–946.

CHAPTER 4. 2001–2013: THE NEW MILLENNIUM

Augustus C. Long Health Sciences Library. Columbia University Medical Center. Records of the Office of the Dean (College of Dental Medicine/Lamster). Archives & Special Collections; 3 boxes.

Graham, R., L. A. Zubiaurre Bitzer, O. R. Anderson, M. Klyvert, L. Moss-Salentijn, and I. B. Lamster. "Advancing the Educational Training of Dental Educators: Review of a Model Program." *Journal of Dental Education* 76, no. 3 (March 2012): 303–310.

Lamster, Ira. "Oral Health Care Services for Older Adults: A Looming Crisis." *American Journal of Public Health* 94, no. 5 (May 2004): 699–702.

Lamster, Ira B., and Mary Northridge, eds. *Improving Oral Health for the Elderly: An Interdisciplinary Approach.* New York: Springer, 2008.

Marshall, S., M. E. Northridge, L. D. De La Cruz, R.D. Vaughan, J. O'Neil-Dunne, and I. B. Lamster. "ElderSmile: A Comprehensive Approach to Improving Oral Health for Seniors." *American Journal of Public Health* 99, no. 4 (April 2009): 595–599.

Mao, J. J., S. G. Kim, J. Zhou, L.Ye, S. Cho, T. Suzuki, S. Y. Fu, R. Yang, and X. Zhou. "Regenerative Endodontics: Barriers and Strategies for Clinical Translation." *Dental Clinics of North America.* 56, no. 3 (July 2012): 639–649.

Tabak, L., and S. Turner. "The Importance of Scientific Research and Teaching Critical Thinking in Academic Dental Institutions: Reactions to Dominic P. DePaola's 'The Revitalization of U.S. Dental Education.'" *Journal of Dental Education* 72, no. 2 supplement (2008): 43–45.

CHAPTER 5: 2014–2016 AND BEYOND: PLANS FOR THE NEXT 100 YEARS

Holiday, Houghton *Dental Columbian,* 1937.

Kac, Mark. "Synoptic Description of Talk Entitled 'Whither Stochastic Processes?'" *SIAM Review* 15, no. 1 (January 1973): 256.

Stohler, C. "State of the College 2014." Accessed September 10, 2015. www.dental-columbia.educ.

Emails on the Curriculum:

- Letty Moss-Salentijn, Vice Dean for Curriculum Innovation and Interprofessional Education: June 6, 2015 and July 29, 2015
- Louis Mandel, Associate Dean for Extramural Hospital Programs: June 1, 2015
- Kavita Ahluwalia, Associate Professor of Dental Medicine: July 21, 2015
- Richard Lichtenthal, Chair Section of Adult Restorative Dentistry: May 28, 2015

- Panos Papapanou, Chair Section of Oral and Diagnostic Sciences: June 25, 2015
- Sidney Eisig, Chair Section of Hospital Dentistry: June 20, 2015
- Burton Edelstein, Chair Section on Population Oral Health: June 16, 2015

  ○ Joseph McManus, Director of Community DentCare program: June 9, 2015

- Steven Chussid, Chair Section of Growth and Development: June 19, 2015

Other Emails:

- Research: Carol Kunzel, Director of the Office of Research Administration: June 15, 2015
- Urban, Rural and Global Initiatives: Ronnie Myers, Vice Dean for Administration, July 16, 2015

CHAPTER 6. STUDENTS AND ALUMNI

Delany S., and A. E. Delany, with A. Hill Hearth. *Having Our Say: The Delany Sisters' First 100 Years*. New York: Dell/Random House, 1997.

Formicola, Allan J. "Women: A Resource for Dental Education." *New York State Dental Journal* 59 (1993): 39–432.

"*Primus* Notable: Ronald Dubner DDS '58, PhD '64." *Primus* (Fall 2005): inside back cover page.

"*Primus* Notable: Paul N. Baer '45, Perio '55." *Primus* (Summer 2010): back cover.

"*Primus* Notable: Dana Graves '80." *Primus* (Summer 2009): back cover.

Journal of the William Jarvie Society 56 (Spring 2013): 16.

Dean's Annual Reports, 1928–1963. Available Augustus C. Long Library, Archives and Special Collections, Columbia University Medical Center, NY.

Central Files: School of Dental and Oral Surgery Alumni Records 1917–1990

Box 1:

- Report of the President of the Alumni Association on Fund-Raising 1979–80.

Box 2:

- January 5, 1940 letter to James Dunning from C.E. Lovejoy regarding special committee on alumni of the College of Dental and Oral Surgery
- Dean's Day Program sponsored by the Dental Alumni, January 28, 1949

Box 3:

- Program for the 25th anniversary of the Dental Hygiene Program, 1937

Index

hospital dentistry section, 165–67
hospitals: affiliation with, 7, 63–64; hospital-university partnership, 7; oral and maxillofacial surgery and hospital dentistry, 104–6; residency programs, 103–4. *See also* specific hospitals
Howard University, 55
Hoyt, Earle, 47
Hughes, Anna, 38, 39, 246
Hunter College, 37, 107
Hurricane Sandy, 150

Ibsen, Olga, 236, 237
Implant Center, 164
implant dentistry. *See* dental implants
Implantology Center, 146
Improving Oral Health for the Elderly (Lamster and Northridge), 127
income, 33, 50, 76
Indian Health Service, 174
infirmary fees, 50
insufficient facilities, 64–65
internal review, 153–57
International Association of Dental Research, 10
internships, 53
interprofessional education, 159
Isabella Geriatric Center, 126, 132, 159
Ivahoe, Herman, 235, 237

Jackson, Lois, 203, 234, 236, 237
Jacobs, William, 235, 237
Jaffe, Margot, 192–94, 234, 236, 237, 240
James Winston Benfield Associate Professor, 160
Japan, 128
Jarvie, James, 8
Jarvie, William, 8, 17, 40, 186, 188
Jerome L. Green Science Center, 173

John F. Kennedy High School, 169
Johns Hopkins Medical Center, 7
Josephs, Elias, 102, 103
Josephs, Philip, 102, 103
Josephs, Saleem, 101, 102–3
Joskow, Renee, 243
Josza, David, 233
Journal of Dental Research, 10
Journal of the Allied Dental Societies, 10
Journal of the American Dental Association, 72
Journal of the William Jarvie Society, 186–87, 188
Judy, Kenneth W.M., 233

Kahn, Norman, 81, 95, 96
Kamen, Paul, 40
Kamen, Saul, 40
Karabin, Susan, 132, 197
Karlan, Frances, 235, 237
Karshan, Max, 40
Kaslick, Ralph, 240, 242
Kess, Steven, 176, 233
Kids International Dental Service, 174
Kim, Martin (Sahng Gyoon), 164
Kim, Syngcuk, 240, 242
King Saud University, 171
Kirk, Grayson, 61, 64, 65
Kittay, Irving, 40
Klyvert, Marlene, 100, 112, 140, 181
Knishkowy, Emanuel, 40
Koch, Edward, 115
Koch, Robert, 43
Koussow, Victor, 33–34, 36, 221
Kramer, Sidney, 29
Krizek, Thomas, 104
Kucine, Allan, 242
Kudler, George, 235
Kulick, Arthur, 235, 237
Kunzel, Carol, 172, 223, 229

New York State, 48, 56, 73

New York State Academic Dental
Centers, 132

New York State capitation aid, 73, 75,
85–86

New York State Dental Foundation, 132

New York Times, 52, 57

New York University, 124, 155

Nicholas, Stephen, 174

NIDCR. *See* National Institute of
Dental and Craniofacial Research
(NIDCR)

night bottle caries, 42

NIH. *See* National Institutes of Health

ninetieth anniversary gala, 132, *134*

Northern Manhattan Community
Voices Collaborative (NMCVC), 116

Northridge, Mary, 127

Nougerole, Zoila, *134*, 147

Novakovic, Gordana Vunjak, 166

"Oath for the Oral Health
Professions," 150

Ochsenbein, Cliff, 191

Office of Diversity and Multicultural
Affairs, 137

Office of Education and Behavioral
Science, 68

Ofner, Henrietta, 178

O'Grady, George, 235

Oh, Daniel, 154, 166, 225–26

OKU, 35

older adults. *See* geriatric oral health care

Oman, Carl, 35, 57

operative dentistry division, 123, 160

Oppie McCall, John, 25

oral and diagnostic sciences section,
163–65

oral and maxillofacial surgery division,
97, 123, 163, 165–66

oral and maxillofacial surgery
residency, 104–6

oral biology division, 123, 163

oral diagnosis, 72

oral disease interaction research,
229–31

oral pathology division, 123

oral surgery advanced courses, 53

oral surgery division, 51, 105

orientation program, 186

Orland, Frank J., 13

orofacial growth and development
division, 71

oropharyngeal cancer research, 223–24

orthodontia, 32

orthodontics division, 51, 123,
147, *149*, 170

Osaka Dental University, 128

Outstanding Vision-Academic Dental
Institution Award, 135, *135*

Owre, Alfred, 2, 4, *18*, 18–24, *21*, 31, 32,
33, 39, 41, 54, 61, 79, 100, 201, 245

Pagonis, Tom, 199

"Painless Parker", 6

pain research, 226–27

Panagakos, Fotinos S., 233

Papapanou, Panos, 94, 139, 154, *161*, 163,
164, *187*, 230–31

Pardes, Herbert, 88, 120–21

pass/fail system of grading, 204–5

Pataki, George, 124

pathophysiology course, 96–97

Pathways to the Future campaign, 197

Patricia McLean Dental Hygiene
Symposium, 195

Patterson, Sara, 81, *82*

Pedersen, Paul O., 42

pediatric dentistry, 54

pediatric dentistry clinic, 29